DR MALCOLM KENDRICK

A Statin Nation

Damaging Millions in a Brave
New Post-Health World

First published in the UK by John Blake Publishing
an imprint of Bonnier Books UK
4th Floor, Victoria House
Bloomsbury Square,
London, WC1B 4DA
England

Owned by Bonnier Books
Sveavägen 56, Stockholm, Sweden

www.facebook.com/johnblakebooks ❶
twitter.com/jblakebooks ❷

First published in paperback in 2018

Paperback ISBN: 978-1-78606-825-5
Ebook ISBN: 978-1-78946-025-4

British Library Cataloguing-in-Publication Data:

A catalogue record for this book is available from the British Library.

Design by www.envydesign.co.uk

Printed and bound in Great Britain by Clays Ltd, Elcograf S.p.A

3 5 7 9 10 8 6 4

Illustrations by Becky Sidwell (bexboo18@googlemail.com)

Text and illustrations ©Malcolm Kendrick 2018

The right of Malcolm Kendrick to be identified as the author of this work has been asserted by him in accordance with the Copyright, Designs and Patents Act 1988.

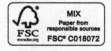

John Blake Publishing is an imprint of Bonnier Books UK
www.bonnierbooks.co.uk

A Statin Nation

Malcolm Kendrick was born and brought up in Scotland, where his father taught him to treat all 'experts' with a degree of scepticism, highlighted by ripping out a page from a school textbook and announcing it was 'rubbish'. He graduated from Aberdeen University and now practices as a GP in Cheshire. He married the lovely Nikki, who taught him never to get ahead of himself: 'All other people are not idiots, you know.' He has two children, Katie, who is studying medicine in Cardiff, and Luke, who is currently a teacher in London. They both look up to him in awe . . . wondering how such a complete technological numbskull could ever have got this far without complete disaster. Malcolm has been studying heart disease for many years, publishing, speaking and writing the occasional book on the matter, including his bestselling *The Great Cholesterol Con* (John Blake Publishing, 2007). He feels that, at some point, the world will finally realise that the cholesterol hypothesis is nonsense, but this may not be in his lifetime. He has his Nobel prizewinning speech ready, however, just in case.

Contents

Introduction

Almost ten years ago, I wrote a book called *The Great Cholesterol Con*. I tried to outline, as clearly as I could, why the central ideas about cardiovascular disease (CVD, i.e. basically heart attacks and strokes) were absolutely, completely and totally wrong. I knew that the impact would be instant and earth shattering.

There would be an immediate realisation that saturated fat and cholesterol have nothing whatsoever to do with CVD. Medical experts and opinion leaders would reverse their thinking, and the public would fling their statins into the nearest dustbin. Guidelines would be hastily rewritten around the world. My Nobel Prize would be polished furiously in Sweden. My acceptance speech was already written and it was a cracker ... humble, witty, incisive.

History reveals that it hasn't quite worked out that way. It is true that, over the last ten years, the guidelines have been rewritten, but they now advise that hundreds of millions *more* people need to be put on statins, at ever-lower levels of blood cholesterol. Furthermore, people have never been more terrified of having a high cholesterol level than today. Supermarket shelves groan under the weight of low-fat foods, designed to lower cholesterol. Benecol sales seem to be going through the roof, rather than down the drain. I think it would be true to say that the 'Cholesterol hypothesis' has never been more potent than now.

Oh well. Perhaps I should rewrite the ending of the story about the emperor's new clothes ... 'So perfectly had everyone allowed themselves to be fooled, that even when the little boy shouted "but he isn't wearing any clothes" the crowd just turned on him, and told him to shut up and stop being so stupid. The End.'

Undeterred, I am having another go, despite the fact that insanity has been defined as doing the same thing again and again while expecting a different result. (And before you say that's an Einstein quote, check it out on *Wikipedia*.) Perhaps I just need to shout a bit louder and carry a baseball bat to be used at good strategic moments.

In truth, over the last ten years many things have changed. Some for the better, some for the worse. Of course, whether you think things are better or worse rather depends on which side of the argument you are on.

Prescribing statins has continued to rise inexorably, with the latest recommendations in the UK being that every single man should be taking a statin by the age of sixty, regardless of whether they have any other risk factors for CVD. The official ceremony when you 'reach the age of lifelong statination' is significantly younger in the US, as you might expect.

Looking at this latest development from a different angle, it is now possible to have 'perfect' cholesterol levels, 'perfect' blood pressure and 'perfect' every other single risk factor, yet when you reach a certain age the danger of suffering a cardiovascular (CV) event is so frighteningly high that you will have to take a drug, every day, for the rest of your life. (An event is a heart attack, stroke or hospital admission with angina, or suchlike.) Of course, hardly anyone has perfect risk factors, which means that the average age when a man is required to take a statin is about fifty, and about ten years later for women.

'And lo, it came to pass that all of the peoples in the world, past middle age, hast been defined as having a new medical condition that shalt be called "statin deficiency syndrome" (SDS).' By order of the management. In other words, your cholesterol level can be low, medium or high, but the actual figure does not matter a jot, you still need a statin to lower it further. This remains true, even if your cholesterol level is lower than that found in any population in the world, even it if is lower than 99.99 per cent of anyone currently alive.

We now live in the 'upside down', a world where there is no cholesterol level that cannot benefit from being lower. A world where cholesterol can cause CVD, even when it is abnormally low. Try and pick the logic out of that, my friend. And if you do, please let me know how you did it.

If things continue their inexorable direction, the next argument – which is already being made – is that CVD gradually develops with ageing. Ergo, you should really start taking statins when you are a child. My prediction is that it will soon be recommended that everyone starts 'statination' in their early twenties, and must continue ... forever. You read it here first. Then we truly will have a 'statin nation' instead of the rather pathetic 14 million statin takers we now have. Or at least are supposed to have. In truth, a lot of people don't take them, even when they tell the doctor that they do.

And in addition to the 'statination' of the entire adult population, we now have ever lower limits for treating blood pressure. About thirty years ago, hypertension was diagnosed if you had blood pressure of over 160/110mmHg. As with cholesterol levels, this target has fallen and fallen. At the time of writing we have reached 130/80mmHg, which means just about everybody has it.

Simultaneously, the concept of pre-hypertension has gained traction. Pre-hypertension means that you don't have blood pressure quite high enough to be diagnosed as hypertension, but you are nearly there and, as is the way of things, you will inevitably become hypertensive. Ergo, you might as well start taking drugs to lower your blood pressure now.

What else? We have a new medical condition known as pre-diabetes. A state of having a highish blood sugar level, but not actually high enough to be diagnosed as diabetes, at least not until they lower the diagnostic threshold once more. However, my friend, bad luck, you *will* inevitably develop diabetes over time so you might as well start the medications now.

Osteoporosis (thinning of bones), is something that women tend to get more than men, and if you have it you must start taking drugs for the rest of your life. These drugs (such as alendronic acid or risedronate) are usually called bisphosphonates and, as an added bonus, you will also take a calcium supplement and vitamin D at the same time.

But that's far from the end. In the same way that we now have pre-hypertension, pre-diabetes and the inexorable lowering of cholesterol levels, there has been pressure to further widen the market for osteoporosis drugs. This has led to the creation of a new condition called osteopenia, which means thinnish bones, not quite osteoporosis, but getting there. Pre-osteoporosis, if you like. So, guess what, time to start the medications to thicken up the old bones. To be taken forever, for the rest of your life. And you may have noticed a certain trend here ...

Now, heart disease. Whilst you're religiously taking statins, you might as well take an aspirin to add further protection. But aspirin can damage the lining of your stomach, so you should also take an anti-acid drug, such as omeprazole, to prevent this, which gives you two more drugs to take – for the rest of your life. Then, if you are unlucky enough to have had an episode of chest pain, which might or might not have been related to your heart, there are a whole load of other drugs that you will be put on for the rest of your life. An ACE-inhibitor, a beta blocker, clopidogrel, etc. It doesn't much matter if the pain seemed cardiac, you can't be too careful you know.

So today, without really trying and without having any disease diagnosed, you can be on at least eleven drugs. Two to lower blood sugar, two blood pressure lowering drugs, aspirin, omeprazole, alendronic acid, the calcium/vitamin D combination, clopidogrel and a statin. In fact, in one of the places where I work I've toyed with the idea of getting a large stamp with a list of these drugs imprinted on it. This will save me the time of writing them out for every single bloody patient who comes to my surgery. Just a quick whack on the prescription ... all drugs present and correct, sir.

The simple fact is that the medical world that has emerged

in the last ten years is not just a statin nation. It is, in my view, a completely bonkers, over-medicated nation. (I did not feel that this might be such a catchy title for the book but, you never know ...) And is all this a good thing? A 2017 Cambridge University study on the increasing use of medications revealed that:

- Almost half of the over-65s in England are taking at least five different drugs a day
- Some were taking up to 23 tablets every day (and I've have known them take far more)
- The proportion taking no pills at all is just 7 per cent
- Heart disease pills, such as statins, accounted for nearly half the medicines taken
- Taking up to five tablets a day increased the danger of premature death by an estimated 47 per cent
- Those taking six medicines or more a day were nearly three times as likely to die prematurely[1]

In fact long ago, when I was a medical student, we were told that no one should be on more than five medications, due to potentially damaging drug interactions, etc. The harms would overwhelm any benefits. Today ... prescribe five drugs minimum or you are not really trying. 'An undermedicated patient ... off with his doctor's head!'

Some voices protest at this dystopian brave new world, and there is now a growing movement called Too Much Medicine supported by medical journals and an increasing number of doctors. The basic theme is, 'Can we stop prescribing so many damned drugs – please. And can we also stop, or at least reduce, all this screening and monitoring and measuring.'

Unfortunately, although I view this movement with benign approval, I rate its chances of success as equal to that of King Canute (now, rather disappointingly, called King Knut) in holding back the tide. Most people, it seems, love to take drugs and submit themselves to every possible screening test known to man. You cannot be too careful, you know. Oh yes, you can.

Most doctors love to prescribe drugs. It gives them something to do, I suppose, and is the fastest way of getting patients out of the surgery. Furthermore, the major medical societies, the experts, the guideline writers, those advising governments around the world want more, more and even more medicine. And so, to no one's great surprise, do the pharmaceutical companies.

I can see the attraction. Pop a few pills and all your health concerns simply disappear. Don't bother to exercise, continue to work far too many hours, drink far too much and relegate good personal relationships to a waste of precious time. Never mind ... all health problems are banished if you swallow a few pills every day. Good luck with that, my friend.

A more recent phenomenon, which has grown rapidly alongside mass medication, is the highly contentious and censorious world of nutrition. Eat this, don't eat that and absolutely never, EVER eat that ... Fortunes are made promoting various, completely mad diets. People used to eat pretty much what they liked but, in the last decade or so, nutrition has become a battleground with various foods becoming the enemy, feared and distrusted. Food has always been an emotive issue with different foods being viewed as good and bad, but there has never been a time of such unrestrained warfare.

Whilst writing this introduction, a documentary was released by Netflix called 'What the Health'. The programme reported various claims, including:

- The World Health Organisation (WHO) has classified bacon and sausage as carcinogenic to humans, on the same level as smoking
- Eating one egg a day is as bad as smoking five cigarettes a day
- The risk of heart disease is 50 per cent for meat eaters, 45 per cent for vegetarians and 4 per cent for vegans
- One serving of processed meat a day increases risk of developing diabetes by 51 per cent

I must remember to warn my pussycat to stop eating so much meat, but he doesn't seem keen on vegetables. I have no doubt that these claims are the purest, refined, organic baloney. Equally, according to The Times this documentary cited two pro-vegan organisations among its frequently listed sources,.

It is true to say that similar warnings about a range of foodstuffs are unnervingly common. The American Heart Association (AHA) majestically proclaimed a 'Presidential Advisory on Harms of Saturated Fat'. Commenting on it David Katz, MD, director of the Yale University Prevention Research Center, and founder and president of the True Health Initiative described the new AHA advisory as 'one of the most important papers addressing the topic of saturated fat and health outcomes'. He added, 'The conclusion is perfectly clear and entirely decisive: saturated fat from the usual dietary sources increases the risk of heart disease, and its replacement with wholesome foods and unsaturated fats reduces that risk.'[2]

I nearly choked on my cornflakes. Except, of course, I do not eat cornflakes because they taste of nothing and are instantly converted to sugar in your digestive system. My breakfast of choice is full fat Greek yoghurt with walnuts and honey. Failing that, bacon, eggs and sausages or sometimes a cheese and ham omelet, which is much more difficult to choke on and, as I shall demonstrate, far healthier and less likely to cause CVD. But back to this 'Presidential Advisory'; let's compare it with a Swedish review from 2013, which stated that:

> Butter, olive oil, heavy cream, and bacon are not harmful foods. Quite the opposite. Fat is the best thing for those who want to lose weight. *And there are no connections between a high fat intake and cardiovascular disease.*
>
> On Monday, SBU, the Swedish Council on Health Technology Assessment, dropped a bombshell. After a two-year long inquiry, reviewing 16,000 studies, the report 'Dietary Treatment for Obesity' upends the conventional dietary guidelines for obese or diabetic people.
>
> For a long time, the healthcare system has given the public advice to avoid fat, saturated fat, and calories. A low-carb diet (LCHF – Low Carb High Fat, is actually a Swedish 'invention') has been dismissed as harmful, a humbug and as being a fad diet lacking any scientific basis.
>
> Instead, the healthcare system has urged diabetics

to eat a lot of fruit (=sugar) and low-fat products with considerable amounts of sugar or artificial sweeteners, the latter a dangerous trigger for the sugar-addicted person.

This report turns the current concepts upside down and advocates a low-carbohydrate, high-fat diet, as the most effective weapon against obesity.[3]

Back and forth the argument goes, with no one listening on either side whilst facts are twisted and manipulated on all sides. I can see this battle going on for another fifty years, at least. Yes, the Lilliputians and Blefuscans do like a pointless war.

If the authorities have failed to make you sufficiently worried about eating fat, you can be made to fear drinking alcohol as well. Years ago, the recommended limits for safe alcohol consumption were 52 units for men and 28 for women, per week. Oh, happy days. However, as with everything else, these limits have tightened and tightened. It is difficult to keep up, but I think we are now down to two units a day as the absolute maximum for men. This issue was reported in *The Guardian*:

> England's chief medical officer has defended tough new drinking guidelines, insisting that the updated advice is not scaremongering but based on 'hard science'. The new recommendation of only 14 units of alcohol, or seven pints of beer, a week means that England now has one of the strictest drinking guidelines in the world.
>
> Dame Sally Davies, the chief medical officer for England, robustly backed the advice in a round of broadcast interviews on Friday, saying that other

countries would follow suit because of new research on the health risks of even moderate drinking.

Speaking on *BBC Breakfast* she said: 'My job as chief medical officer is to make sure we bring the science together to get experts to help us fashion the best low-risk guidelines.

'If you take 1,000 women, 110 will get breast cancer without drinking. Drink up to these guidelines and an extra 20 women will get cancer because of that drinking. Double the guideline limit and an extra 50 women per 1,000 will get cancer. Take bowel cancer in men: if they drink within the guidelines their risk is the same as non-drinking. But if they drink up to the old guidelines an extra 20 men per 1,000 will get bowel cancer. That's not scaremongering, that's fact and it's hard science.' [4]

Anyway, the direction of travel is abundantly clear. Not drinking at all, ever, is 'journey's end' for the experts on alcohol. And not eating saturated fat, ever, is 'journey's end' for our dietary experts. At the same time, new limits for cholesterol, blood pressure, diabetes and suchlike will mean that everyone will be on multiple medications from ever younger ages, with new lifelong drugs being added on a depressingly frequent basis.

Left to their own devices, experts drift inexorably to extremism. After all, what is the point of having an important new guidelines meeting if you can't then tighten, ban, enforce or demand that everyone must do something different. The inevitable end result being either 'nothing' or 'everything'. This is now a well-defined phenomenon of 'group-think', as outlined in this article in the *Spectator*: 'To become an extremist, hang around with people you agree with. Cass Sunstein – co-author of the hugely influential *Nudge* and an adviser to President Obama – unveils his new theory of 'group polarisation', and explains why, when like-minded people spend time with each other, their views become not only more confident but more extreme.[5]

Over the last ten years, I have watched a large branch of medicine heading in a very strange and extreme direction. I had hoped that various guidelines would become so ridiculous, so distanced from reality, science and logic, and anything else that there would be some kind of backlash. But backlash there came none. Not yet, anyway.

I am not the first person to notice the direction of travel. Well over twenty years ago an article appeared in *The New England Journal of Medicine*. It was called 'The Last Well Person' and with remarkable prescience it covered pretty much everything that needs to be said on this matter. I shall quote a couple of passages.

> I have not met a completely well person in months. At this rate, well people will vanish. As with the extinction of any species, there will be one last survivor. My guess is that the extinction will occur sometime in late 1998. Before we can speculate about the last well person, we need to understand what is happening. Why are they vanishing?
>
> The demands of the public for definitive wellness are colliding with the public's belief in a diagnostic system that can find only disease. A public in dogged pursuit of the unobtainable, combining with clinicians whose

tools are powerful enough to fine very small lesions (a lesion is just a damaged, or diseased bit of the body) is a setup of diagnostic excess ...

What is paradoxical about our awesome diagnostic power is that we do not have a test to distinguish a well person from a sick one. Wellness cannot be screened for. There is no substance in blood or urine whose level is reliably low or high in well people. No radiological shadows or images indicated wellness. There is no tissue that can undergo biopsy to prove a person is well.

This magnificent article then goes on to describe the last well person in some detail. A man who has chosen a job with as little stress as possible, living in an area of the US with a mean wind-chill factor, in a temperate range, in January. He has a screening test for blood sugar, cholesterol, carcinoembryonic antigen, prostate specific antigen and occasional stool tests. He did have two unnecessary colonoscopies because of false positive tests for blood in his bowel movement, and now abstains from meat for a week before any stool test. Also ...

He consumes 15 per cent of his calories as fat, with the remainder split between protein and carbohydrates. He completely avoids saturated fat, salt, sugar and red meat, and all but trace amounts of vegetable oil, which he uses in his wok to stir-fry his vegetables. He was a regular eater of tofu until he heard Garrison Keillor say on the radio that Tofu did not extend anyone's useful life, but only that last few weeks in a terminal coma.

Every day he takes vitamins C, E, B₆, and a small amount of D, several doses of kelp; and a concoction of dried seaweed mixed with desalinated sea water, along with a baby aspirin. He takes three doses of bulk laxatives, eats a bowl of bran, and drinks eight glasses of water daily...[6]

Who'd have guessed that this beautifully constructed, somewhat tongue in cheek account of the horribly dystopian lifestyle of the last well man is now almost mainstream behaviour?

Amongst the many doctors I meet, there has been much grumbling about this ever-increasing medicalisation. I regularly hear such phrases as 'bloody monkey medicine'. But those in charge of the medical research complex are highly resistant to any change of direction, and very few people risk popping their heads over the parapet. Dare to challenge the experts and you can expect a vicious reaction.

Fairly recently, a few of us mad cholesterol sceptics were proving more successful than usual in criticising mass statin prescribing. This was *not* to be allowed. One of the big names of cardiology, Professor Steven Nissen, was stung into action. He wrote an article in the *Journal of the American Medical Association* entitled 'Statin Denial: An Internet-Driven Cult With Deadly Consequences', which gives a good sense of the scientific tone of what followed. I presume he felt that his mighty Olympian thunderbolt would keep me, and my fellow cult leaders, firmly in our place. I wish I had known I was running a cult, I could have made some real money.

Tom Naughton, a fellow cholesterol sceptic, writer and humorist, wrote a blog on the Nissen article, and most amusing

14

it was. One of the comments in his article made me laugh and laugh. So, dear reader, I nicked it (with permission):

> You didn't really tell about the worst part of the cult.
>
> Don't forget how cult members are initially recruited with flattery and promises of magnificent rewards in order to get them to pledge nearly all of their family's assets to the cult. Having 'proven worthy,' they are taken to 'education camps' where they are isolated with other recruits and forced to memorise and recite back the cult doctrines. Access to outside information or perspectives is forbidden, and any questioning is swiftly met with threats of ostracism and expulsion.
>
> Once sufficiently indoctrinated, the recruits are coerced into several years of working long, mind-numbing hours of labor at penury 'wages' – ostensibly for the good of the cult, while the poohbahs at the top enjoy riches and lavish lifestyles.
>
> Oh wait. Wrong cult. That's the 'medical school/internships programs' cult.
>
> Never mind. My bad.
>
> Cheers!

And a very powerful cult it is too.

Anyway, where was I? Oh yes, explaining that medicine is heading towards an extreme place that is in danger of damaging us all. Health is not the lowering of numbers on a blood test, nor endless scanning and screening in a desperate attempt to find perfect health. It is a very different thing indeed. Positive mental attitude, for one.

In fact, the WHO, in its very first meeting, stated that health is 'a state of complete physical, mental, and social well-being and not merely the absence of disease or infirmity.' Absolutely true. Most of which has very little to do with the medical profession.

I would also argue that almost all of what we now call 'preventive medicine' has nothing to do with prevention at all. Detecting high blood pressure, for example, is not prevention. It is just finding a problem at an early stage. Cancer screening, again, is not prevention. It is just finding the problem at an early stage. Screening is not preventing.

Moreover, lowering blood pressure is doing nothing for the underlying disease process. You are just lowering a measurement that may or may not be very helpful. Indeed, some anti-hypertensives have been found to lower blood pressure very effectively, yet increase the risk of CVD death.[7]

The same phenomenon of simply lowering numbers has also been found in the world of diabetes. The ACCORD Study, using multiple interventions to lower the blood sugar in people with diabetes, as far as possible, found that this had no effect on CV mortality, but significantly increased overall mortality (overall mortality = the risk of dying of anything): 'As compared with standard therapy, the use of intensive therapy to target normal glycated hemoglobin levels for 3.5 years increased mortality and did not significantly reduce major cardiovascular events. These findings identify a previously unrecognised harm of intensive glucose lowering in high-risk patients with type 2 diabetes.'[8]

More recently, the findings of ACCORD were confirmed by another study that made exactly the same point. Namely, that the more you lower the blood sugar level with drugs, the greater risk of death. Insulin was fingered as the most damaged drug of all. 'The pattern of mortality risk across levels of HbA1c (long term measure of blood sugar levels) differed by glucose-lowering regimen. Lower HbA1c was associated with increased mortality risk compared with moderate control.'[9]

Finding things that are 'wrong' and then attempting to batter them back down to 'normal' does not necessarily end well. Instead, we have been fitted to what I call the 'Procrustean bed of medicine'.

'In the Greek myth, Procrustes was a son of Poseidon with a stronghold on Mount Korydallos at Erineus, on the sacred way between Athens and Eleusis. There he had a bed, in which he invited every passer-by to spend the night, and where he set to work on them with his smith's hammer, to stretch them to fit. In later tellings, if the guest proved too tall, Procrustes would amputate the excess length; nobody ever fitted the bed exactly – so they died.'[10]

Clever people those Greeks.

I believe that we need to move away from defining more and more people as ill, then chopping or stretching things back to 'normal'. Instead we need to move towards 'a state of complete physical, mental, and social well-being'.

I cannot cover everything, but I want to try to help people understand CVD. I will outline the current ideas and explain as well as I can, in some detail, where these ideas have gone wrong, and will sign off by trying to outline the most important things that you can do to maintain good CV health. But before getting into the guts of the matter, I must add that I am not attacking conventional Western medicine. This has been, in many ways, a spectacular success with hip replacements, antibiotics, anesthetics, the treatment of major trauma and the prevention of many diseases that have been a scourge of humanity for millennia. Smallpox, syphilis, polio. Dentistry, new heart valves, painkillers, orthopaedic surgery ... I could go on and on.

However, in CVD prevention, medicine has grabbed the wrong end of the stick and then rushed off, with grim determination, in the wrong direction. I intend to change things round, then the experts can rush back madly from whence they came and head off in the right, damned direction. No offence, guys. Well, not much.

CHAPTER 1

What is CVD?

B efore starting with more exciting topics, such as what causes heart attacks and strokes – and what doesn't – there is the unfortunate requirement of attempting to make clear what I am talking about. A recurring theme in this book is that medical terminology is often hopelessly confusing. It can act as a barrier rather than an aid to understanding. So, here is my initial attempt to attain some form of clarity.

This book is primarily focused on two often fatal conditions – heart attacks and strokes. Whilst there are many different diseases that can damage the heart and the brain, in the majority of cases the problem is a disease of the arteries supplying blood to these organs.

With heart attacks, the arteries affected are the coronary arteries. The disease is often referred to as coronary artery disease (CAD). Other common terms regularly, confusingly and interchangeably used are coronary heart disease (CHD) or ischaemic heart disease (IHD) (ischaemia is a general term that means lack of blood supply, leading to lack of oxygen supply). CAD, CHD and IHD are different terms for describing the same thing.

With strokes, the main problem is with the carotid arteries that supply blood to the brain. These arteries branch from the aorta, the single artery that leaves the heart. The carotid arteries separate from the aorta around the base of the neck. One carotid artery goes up the left side of the neck, the other goes up the right. (There are also vertebral arteries going into the back of your brain, through the spinal column, but they are less likely to cause problems, though they can.)

Whilst the underlying cause of a stroke, as with a heart attack, is disease in the carotid arteries, you will never come across the term carotid artery disease, carotid brain disease or even ischaemic brain disease. Why? That is just the way it is. Equally, I have never heard anyone refer to a stroke as a form of 'brain disease'. It is funny how thinking and terminology, even in closely related areas, can develop in completely different ways.

The actual disease in the blood vessels that leads to most heart attacks and strokes is usually referred to as atherosclerosis. This is the development of lumps, or thickenings, in the artery wall. These thickenings are most often called atherosclerotic plaques.

You may have come across the term arteriosclerosis. I have never worked out what this is, and I don't think anyone else has either. I think it is the same thing as atherosclerosis, even though some people say it is not. So, I will just leave this to one side.

Atherosclerosis, or atherosclerotic plaques, do not just

occur in the coronary and carotid arteries. You can suffer from atherosclerosis in arteries almost anywhere else in the body. Arteries that supply the kidneys, the bowel, liver, adrenal glands ... I recently admitted a lady with severe abdominal pain who had suffered a 'bowel attack'. An artery supplying blood to a section of her large bowel had blocked off completely and her bowel infarcted (infarction is the sudden loss of blood supply due to a blockage, usually a blood clot, leading to death of the downstream tissue). About 0.6 metres of bowel was later removed surgically. I hate to admit it, but I got the diagnosis completely wrong. On the plus side, at least I sent her to hospital, recognising that she wasn't very well. I thought she had bowel cancer and had obstructed.

In short, the underlying disease that we are looking at with heart attacks and strokes is actually vascular disease, which can manifest itself in almost all organs of the body. Vascular disease, due to atherosclerosis, often comes under the umbrella of CVD. This can be shortened to CV, as in CV (cardiovascular) mortality.

I think I also need to explain a bit more about the vascular system. Essentially, this consists of the heart, the arteries and the veins. The heart begins life where an artery and vein merge together. This area then enlarges, develops valves and an electrical conduction system, etc., transforming itself into the fully formed and highly complex organ that we call the heart.

It is the first organ in the body to function, and it starts pushing blood around the body twenty days after conception. As with most aspects of foetal development it is just unbelievable how it happens, and *that* it happens, almost perfectly. Mind-boggling.

The heart pumps blood into the arteries at relatively high

pressure. Veins bring blood back to the heart at much lower pressure. Arteries have much thicker and more muscular walls than veins, primarily because they need to withstand much higher blood pressure. The other main difference between arteries and veins is that the bigger veins have valves in them to stop the blood simply dropping back down to your ankles. If a valve in your leg gives way, you can end up with a bulging varicose vein because of gravity, and increased pressure acting on the vein beneath the failed valve.

Apart from these small differences, arteries and veins have an identical structure. There is a single layer of cells that lines the inner surface. This layer is usually referred to as the endothelium, made of single endothelial cells, which are wide and flat, a bit like miniature wall tiles, although the endothelium can be several cells thick in certain places. Underneath the endothelium there is a muscular/elastic layer, the media. Surrounding the media is a tough outer layer, the adventitia, which holds everything together.

When arteries branch and become smaller and smaller, they are called arterioles. Smaller veins are the venules and the smallest blood vessels are capillaries, which join the arterioles to the venules. These are so narrow that red blood cells must be squashed and distorted in order to squeeze through.

A little-known fact (little known to most doctors I have spoken to, anyway), is that the larger arteries and veins have their own blood vessels to supply them. They are the vasa vasorum, which means blood vessel of the blood vessels. Yes, blood vessels need their own blood vessels to get the nutrients they need. Something I never learned at medical school, for sure; or maybe I was asleep during that lecture.

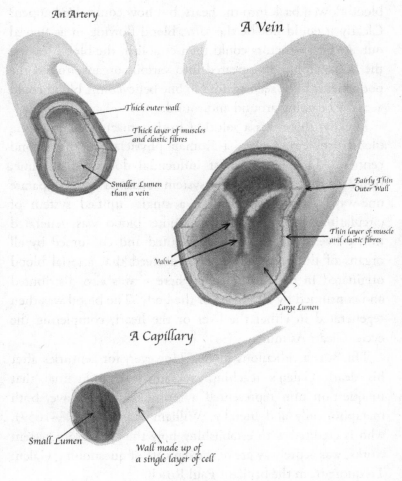

An Artery

A Vein

Thick outer wall

Thick layer of muscles
and elastic fibres

Smaller Lumen
than a vein

Fairly Thin
Outer Wall

Thin layer of muscle
and elastic fibres

Valve

Large Lumen

A Capillary

Small Lumen

Wall made up of
a single layer of cell

DIAGRAM 1

As capillaries are far too small to see with the naked eye, for
many hundreds of years the circulatory system was a bit of
a mystery to everyone. Blood flowed out of the heart, and

blood flowed back into the heart, but how could this happen? Clearly it could not be the same blood flowing in as flowed out. As far as doctors could then establish, the blood leaving the heart simply disappeared into various organs around the body, never to be seen again. No one believed the blood could actually be going around and round.

Luckily, there was a solution to the amazing disappearing blood problem. Galen, a Roman physician in the second century AD, and the most influential doctor of all time, proposed that the circulatory system consisted of two separate one-way systems, rather than a single, unified system of circulation. He thought that venous blood was generated in the liver, and was then distributed and consumed by all organs of the body. He further decreed that arterial blood originated in the heart, from where it was also distributed and consumed by all organs of the body. The blood was then regenerated in either the liver or the heart, completing the cycle. Clear? As mud.

This was a ridiculous model. However, for centuries after his death Galen's teachings remained so influential that to question him represented a terminal career move, both metaphorically and literally. William Harvey (1578–1657), who is credited with establishing how the circulatory system works, was acutely aware of the dangers of questioning Galen. To quote from the brilliant Paul Rosch.

> It is impossible to overestimate the power that Galen had over medicine at the time. He was such an unquestioned authority that he was referred to as 'The Medical Pope of the Middle Ages'. Although Harvey announced his discovery in 1615, he waited 13 years

before publishing his results, since it was considered sacrilegious to challenge Galen.

Any contrary opinions were considered to be heretical, and would not only quickly end your career, but could even cause you to be burned at the stake. Harvey's hesitation to openly defy Galen proved to be justified.

Most physicians rejected his 1628 book because he could not explain how the arteries and veins met. If organs did not consume blood, how did different part of the body obtain nourishment? If the liver did not make blood from food, where did blood originate? Why was blood blue in veins, but red in arteries? It took two decades for Harvey's colleagues to acknowledge his achievements.[1]

It's a great pleasure of mine, almost a secret vice, to read about the history of influential medical ideas. The passage of time has the great benefit of allowing you to see exactly how and why ideas of the greatest stupidity were so widely believed, and then defended with vigour and venom by the great and the good. At which point, you can draw parallels with the thinking and actions of today. Mentioning no names – yet.

Anyway, it turns out that Galen was wrong and Harvey was right, surprise, surprise. Blood does circulate around the body, travelling from the heart, in arteries, down through arterioles and capillaries, and then back again in venules and veins. How simple everything seems when you know the answer.

One point I need to add here is that the heart also pumps blood through the lungs, where it picks up oxygen and gets rid of carbon dioxide. This means that, in the lungs, blood vessels containing high levels of carbon dioxide are called arteries. On the other hand, blood vessels full of oxygen are called veins. And that's the exact opposite in the rest of the body, just to add to the general confusion.

The arteries and veins in the lungs (pulmonary blood vessels) also have the same basic structure as the blood vessels elsewhere in the body. However, both the arteries and veins here have thin walls, as the blood pressure in the lungs is relatively low.

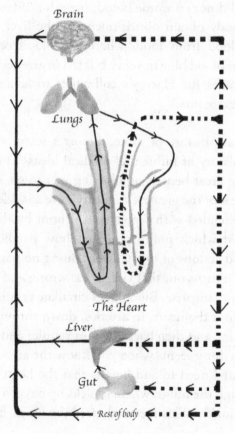

CHAPTER 2

What is the Average Blood Pressure in Various Blood Vessels?

━━━○━━━

For historical reasons, the blood pressure itself is measured using the rather strange units of millimetres of mercury (mmHg – Hg is the shorthand chemical symbol for mercury). That is, how many millimetres of mercury can be pushed up a thin tube by the pressure in the blood vessel. The reason for using mercury is that, historically, it was by far the densest liquid known and, unlike most metals, it is liquid at room temperature.

Mercury is also more than 13 times as dense as water, which means that the column of mercury only needs be one-thirteenth the height of the actual blood pressure you are measuring. If you measure blood pressure using a water sphygmomanometer (the medical name for the blood pressure measuring instrument), it would need to be about 3 metres tall, which is about the height that blood would spurt up if you accidently made a hole in the side of the heart during open heart surgery (do not try this at home). A 3m-long sphygmomanometer would have been a bit inconvenient to carry about in a doctor's bag, and nowadays measuring blood pressure is almost always done electronically with a hand-held machine. How prosaic it has all become. No skill, no blatant guesswork.

The other point to bear in mind is that the blood pressure in the arteries is going up and down all the time. As the heart squeezes (known as systole), the pressure peaks. When the heart relaxes (diastole), the pressure drops. And that's why your blood pressure is normally given in two numbers: systolic (the highest pressure reached) and diastolic (the lowest pressure it falls to, before going up again as the heart contracts).

Normal blood pressure, measured in the arm, is around 120mmHg over 70mmHg and will be recorded in your notes as 120/70. Which of these two figures is more important? Books have been written on the matter but they are not, to tell the truth, very interesting. In general, the systolic pressure is normally considered the most important measurement. I await the inevitable howls of protest on this matter from the 'pointy enders'.

The blood pressure in the coronary arteries is about the same as in the arm, perhaps a little higher. But unlike everywhere else in the body, the blood only flows in the coronary arteries when the heart relaxes (diastole), because when the heart is contracting (systole) the coronary arteries are, in some cases, squeezed shut by the muscle contracting around them.

In veins, however, the blood pressure is very much lower, and does not go up and down with the beating of the heart. It measures around 3–8mmHg, depending on the vein. The blood pressure in pulmonary blood vessels (blood vessels in the lung) is a little higher than in the veins, around 20mmHg over 8mmHg (20/8), i.e. 20mmHg in the pulmonary arteries and 8mmHg in the veins.

The issue of blood pressure in various blood vessels around the body becomes relevant to the entire discussion because (apart from very rare situations), atherosclerosis *never* develops in the veins and only very, very rarely in pulmonary blood vessels. This is even though these blood vessels are exposed to precisely the same concentration of cholesterol as the arteries. Yes, ponder that fact for a few moments.

CHAPTER 3

What is Atherosclerosis?

Atherosclerosis has been described in many ways but, at its simplest, is discrete or patchy thickenings within arterial walls, usually called atherosclerotic plaques. At its most complex, you can read papers discussing seven different types of atherosclerotic plaque, with several subsections in-between. (I remember reading 'A definition of advanced types of atherosclerotic lesions and a histological classification of atherosclerosis' – a report from the committee on vascular lesions of the Council on Arteriosclerosis, the American Heart Association – and ending up none the wiser.)

However you choose to define them, plaques start as small areas, usually described as 'fatty streaks'. Over decades, these streaks grow into bigger and more complex lesions, a lesion being an abnormal/unhealthy thing in the body. At a certain point, they become so big and ugly that they're termed atherosclerotic plaques. I am not sure when a fatty streak becomes a plaque; it's a bit like asking when a boat becomes a ship. Nobody knows.

Plaques, in turn, come in many different versions. Some end up hard and calcified (full of calcium). Others have a gooey, fatty centre, known as a lipid core. If the gooey core is covered by a thin, fibrous cap it will usually be called a vulnerable plaque because, if the cap ruptures, the lipid core will be exposed to the bloodstream and triggers an instant, very large blood clot within the artery. More on this later.

DIAGRAM 3

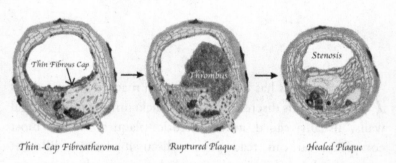

Thin -Cap Fibroatheroma   Ruptured Plaque   Healed Plaque

In general, it is thought that calcified plaques represent the end stage of atherosclerosis plaque development and, slightly counter-intuitively, such plaques are probably stronger, better organised and less likely to rupture than earlier stage plaques. It is the transitional phase, the vulnerable plaque with a lipid core, that is the most dangerous and likely to rupture, leading to disaster.

Over the last few years, a test for measuring calcium in the coronary arteries – the coronary artery calcification (CAC) score – has become popular. The higher score, the more calcium in the artery, thus the more atherosclerotic 'disease' you have and the greater your risk of a heart attack. This assumes that if you have a lot of calcified plaques you will have a lot of other vulnerable, unseen plaques as well.

Unfortunately, you cannot do a great about the calcified plaques. Once they have formed, they have formed, with some caveats. In essence, what you are measuring with a CAC score is your atherosclerotic history – not necessarily your atherosclerotic future. However, if you have no calcium at all in your arteries, you probably have no earlier-stage atherosclerotic disease either, so whatever you were doing, keep doing it.

Four other facts about calcium in your arteries that I find fascinating:

- Statins accelerate calcium build-up in arteries and on heart valves[1]
- You can see considerable calcium deposits in the arteries of mummies from Egypt and other parts of the world
- Warfarin (commonly used in treating atrial fibrillation, or AF – an abnormal heart rhythm) accelerates calcium build-up in arteries, due to its action as a vitamin K antagonist[2]
- There is some reasonably strong evidence that vitamin K supplementation may slow, or possibly even reverse, calcium build-up in arteries

At the risk of going too far off-piste here, in vitamin K supplementation, as with many things to do with vitamins, the mainstream researchers have determinedly tested the wrong form. There are three forms of the vitamin (and probably more, but let's go with three for now): K1, 2 and 3. K1 is often called phylloquinone, which is the one most tested while K3, often called menaquinone, has never been properly tested as a way of preventing or reversing calcification. 'Overall, the available observational population-based evidence, based on dietary intake measures, suggests menaquinone [K3] intake may be more likely to protect against vascular calcification than phylloquinone intake. Yet currently, the only intervention studies have examined the effect of phylloquinone...'[3]

So, observational studies show that K3 is almost certainly the only K vitamin that provides protection but, with wearisome inevitability, it has not been studied in any clinical trial. Only K1 has been used. And this, I am afraid , is typical of mainstream medicine's approach to vitamins. Start by failing to clearly define the 'normal' range of a vitamin – see especially vitamins D and B12, then give a very low dose of the wrong form of the vitamin and then claim that vitamins have no benefits whatsoever – on anything. Do I detect the dead hand of the pharmaceutical industry here?

Once you have done this you can move on to claim that vitamins are dangerous and damaging to health and then, to the sound of distant cheers from all pharmaceutical companies everywhere, ban them. Why? 'Everyone need drugs. Everyone.'

Here is a clue about vitamins. 'Vit' is short for vital, as in vital for health. As in, if you don't get a sufficient amount in your diet, you will die. As in ... well, you get the idea. (Processed foods are often stuffed with synthetic vitamins, the natural ones having been destroyed in the manufacturing process. Oh well.) But more on vitamins later. Let's get back to the main subject: atherosclerosis.

Atherosclerotic plaques are the underlying cause of heart attacks and strokes. They start life as fatty streaks in the middle sections, or media, of the artery walls and grow into plaques. This process starts early. When I say early, I mean early, as it is possible to see thickenings or fatty streaks in the arteries of foetuses within the womb.

The most dangerous phase of plaque development would seem to be the vulnerable plaque which, if it ruptures, can cause a complete blockage in an artery. This can happen in arteries throughout the body but most commonly affects the coronary arteries, which supply blood to the heart, or the carotid arteries, which supply blood to the brain.

CHAPTER 4

Heart Attacks and Strokes

HEART ATTACKS

The heart is supplied with blood by several different coronary arteries, which branch off at regular intervals. Let's say there are four of them – not quite right, but it will do (some people have coronary arteries that others do not possess). The naming system is complex.

All the coronary arteries supply blood to different sections of the heart. The left anterior descending (LAD) artery, for example, supplies blood to the left ventricle that does the heavy lifting of pumping blood out of the aorta at high pressure. The LAD is, therefore, the most 'mission critical' artery in the heart although, obviously, they are all pretty important.

Classically, when you have a heart attack, one of the coronary arteries will suddenly get blocked by a blood clot. This usually happens when a vulnerable plaque ruptures. This, in turn, drastically reduces the blood supply and the area of the heart supplied by that artery can infarct, which is why heart attacks are often called myocardial infarctions (MIs) by the medical profession.

Most textbooks define an infarct as 'death' or 'necrosis' of heart muscle. However, this is simply wrong. It is true that a certain amount of heart muscle affected will die, and the remnants of dead cells will then be cleared away. But, assuming that you survive the MI, a repair process kicks into action to convert heart muscle cells (myocytes) into scar tissue. To repeat, infarction does not represent heart muscle death. Yes, some cells die, but most of them simply stop contracting in a desperate attempt to save energy. These cells are then converted into scar tissue, which requires very little oxygen to survive.

This is a tightly controlled process, ensuring that the basic structure of the heart remains intact. If this did not happen, an infarcted area of the heart would simply disintegrate, which would be instantly fatal. The infarction process was well described in the paper 'Infarct scar – a dynamic tissue':

> Following MI, with loss of necrotic cardiac myocytes [dead heart muscle cells], a reparative process is quickly initiated to rebuild infarcted myocardium [rebuilding the area of heart damaged by sudden blood loss] and maintain structural integrity of the ventricle. A series of cellular responses are called into play driven largely by cell-cell signalling that serves to regulate tissue repair. Initially, inflammatory cells are attracted to and invade the site of injury ... new blood vessels are formed (angiogenesis), and fibroblast-like cells appear and replicate. This early inflammatory phase of healing

with resultant granulation tissue formation is followed
by a fibrogenic phase that eventuates in scar tissue – *a
rebuilding of infarcted myocardium.*[1]

Apologies for the jargon, but I thought it was worthy of full
inclusion as I want you to know that we are most certainly
not looking at a simple, passive process in MI. The infarcted
area does not die. Instead it is reconstructed into scar tissue,
but obviously this area of the heart cannot pump afterwards
as it will be made of passive scar tissue, rather than healthy,
contracting heart muscle cells (myocytes).

Sometimes, after an obstructive blood clot, the heart muscle
does not infarct when the blood supply is lost. Instead, the
affected area of heart muscle simply stops beating and enters
a state known as hibernation. Just like in a hibernating bear,
everything is still turning over, but at a very low rate. So, the
myocytes are still alive but no longer contracting in order to
reduce oxygen demand.

These hibernating areas can spring back to life if the
blood supply improves. Alternatively, they can remain in
hibernation for years, only to fully infarct at some point in
the future, presumably after giving up hope of ever having
enough oxygen to function. In some cases, the heart muscle
does not infarct or hibernate, it simply struggles on, but will
protest loudly if you try to exercise. This painful protest
is called angina. Angina can also develop when a coronary
artery gradually narrows over time, and is often called
ischaemic (from ischaemia, meaning lack of oxygen) heart
disease (IHD).

At one time, it was thought that if a coronary artery was
fully blocked, this would inevitably lead to death. However,

in 1912 an American doctor called Herrick became the first to describe an arterial blockage, without the patient dying. A non-fatal MI.

Since that initial observation, it has been increasingly recognised that many MIs are not fatal. Indeed, in many cases people are completely unaware that they have even had an MI. Whilst the classic heart attack is described as someone clutching at their chest, in agony, with pain going down the left arm and up into the jaw, sweating and pale, this is not always the case.

'If the patient has no symptoms or atypical symptoms, the MI may be categorised as "silent". In some (but not all) cases, silent MI may be later identified and referred to as "unrecognised MI". Unrecognised MI is a common and clinically significant event.'[2]

How can it be that some MIs result in agonising, crushing pain, whilst other MIs are silent? Frankly, I have no idea, but silent MIs are more common in women, the elderly and people who have other, underlying conditions, e.g. diabetes. That doesn't explain why they are silent. It is just an observation.

To complicate things even further, you can find people with symptomatic MIs, ECG (heart trace) changes that are indicative of an MI, and raised cardiac enzymes that are all fully diagnostic of an MI, where no blockage of any artery can be found. This is known as myocardial infarction with non-obstructed coronary arteries (MINOCA). This can represent up to 25 per cent of MIs. And in addition to these variants, it is fully possible for a blood clot to form in a completely non-atherosclerotic artery and go on to cause an MI. This is relatively uncommon, but does happen.

Finally, for now, although I could go on far longer if I

included all possible forms of heart attack, you can have Takotsubo syndrome. This has almost all the signs of a classic MI: chest pain, breathlessness, collapse, raised cardiac enzymes and ECG changes, etc., and you can even die of it. Yet there is no blood clot, no area of infarction and no true MI at all. This is sometimes called broken heart syndrome and is usually brought on by sudden, emotional stress. The Japanese were the first to recognise this phenomenon, and so named it because the left ventricle (the main pumping chamber of the heart) changes shape and ends up looking like an octopus pot – a *takotsubo*. You mean you didn't know what a Japanese octopus pot looks like?

Well, the left ventricle ends up looking like an octopus pot anyway, Which proves something that I have banged on about for years, namely that human emotions have a significant impact on physical health – and, of course, vice versa. More later.

DIAGRAM 4

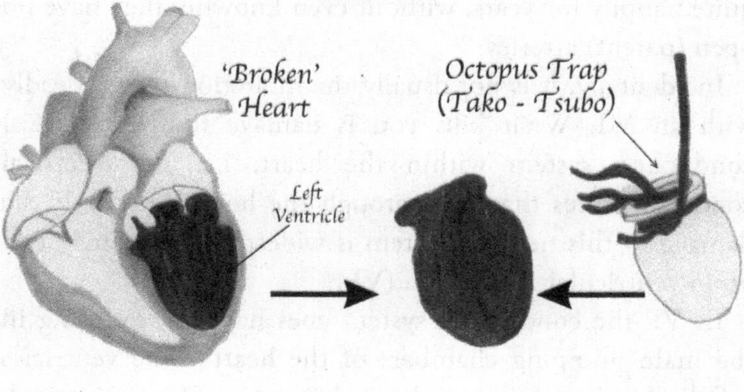

'Broken' Heart

Octopus Trap (*Tako - Tsubo*)

Left Ventricle

Whilst there are many different type of heart attack, it remains true that the classic MI is the most common event, and the process is as follows. Over many years, a coronary artery narrows, as the underlying atherosclerotic plaque enlarges. Then the plaque ruptures, leading to the formation of a fully obstructive blood clot. This cuts off blood supply and an infarction will ensue. Around 40 per cent of classic MIs are immediately fatal.

One further complicating factor that I need to mention is that the heart can create new, smaller blood vessels over time known as collateral circulation. If your coronary arteries have been getting more and more blocked, over the years, newly created blood vessels can and will bypass the narrow areas to keep the oxygen supply going. If the collateral circulation is sufficiently well developed, this can fully protect the heart from a blood clot finally blocking a narrowed coronary artery. In some people, all their coronary arteries are completely blocked yet they can still function well. Indeed, they can live quite happily for years, without even knowing they have no open (patent) arteries.

Incidentally, it is not usually the infarction that is deadly with an MI. What kills you is damage to the electrical conduction system within the heart, i.e. the electrical condition fibres that run through the heart muscle. If the damage to this nervous system is widespread, you may end up in ventricular fibrillation (VF).

In VF the conduction system goes haywire, resulting in the main pumping chambers of the heart – the ventricles – failing to beat in a coordinated manner. They just twitch and spasm as electrical impulses fire about all over the place. This reduces blood flow to zero which, in turn, leads quite rapidly to death. If someone goes into VF, it can be possible to shock the heart back into its normal rhythm using a defibrillator. They are now found everywhere, even in remote telephone boxes, gyms and libraries. This is an excellent scheme because, from the onset of VF, you have about four to five minutes to act before the lack of oxygen supply to the brain leads to irreversible damage. So, the sooner you can shock someone back into normal rhythm, the better.

Luckily, modern defibrillators can virtually talk you through the process. You switch them on, stick the pads on the chest, stand back and they know what to do. They will recognise if someone is in VF or not, and shock accordingly. You become a mere bystander. However, if there is no electrical activity at all, giving a flat-line on the ECG, the defibrillator cannot work as there is no activity to restore. In this case cardio pulmonary resuscitation (CPR) is the only way to keep someone alive for long enough to get the person to hospital in time. At which point, other more complicated matters can be attempted. But bear in mind that well-performed CPR can keep people alive for hours – so please *don't stop* when you get tired or disheartened.

In the immediate aftermath of an MI, assuming you are not in VF, and assuming you are not already dead, once you reach the hospital many different things can now happen. You could simply be given an aspirin, which slows or stops blood clots from forming. In fact, you probably will already have been given one. You might also be given a clot buster, such as tissue plasminogen activator (tPA). This converts plasminogen, an inactive substance incorporated into all blood clots, into plasmin. Plasmin rapidly slices blood clots apart, through an action called fibrinolysis. Fibrin consists

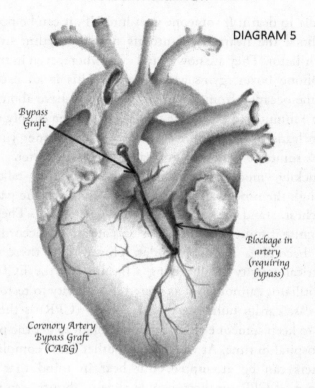

DIAGRAM 5

Bypass Graft

Blockage in artery (requiring bypass)

Coronary Artery Bypass Graft (CABG)

of long, sticky stands of protein that bind blood clots tightly together. Fibrinolysis makes the clots disintegrate. Alternatively, you could have an emergency bypass graft operation. This is where veins are stripped out of your leg and used to bypass the blockage in the artery in your heart.

However, these activities are now considered somewhat 'five minutes ago'. Nowadays, the most common treatment is percutaneous coronary intervention (PCI), when a thin probe is inserted into an artery in your arm or leg. It is then cunningly directed into the blocked coronary artery, whereupon a balloon will be inflated to widen the artery. At which point, in most cases, a metal lattice framework that has been wrapped around the balloon is opened out. This provides a rigid structure to keep the artery fixed open after the balloon has been deflated and pulled back out. This is called a stent and the procedure stenting. After this you will be put on a cocktail of different drugs to take for the rest of your life ... But that is a different story.

It must be said that the treatment of an MI has improved beyond all recognition. In the bad old days, the only treatment following an MI was pain relief and a stern instruction to lie immobile in bed for six weeks, during which time the heart muscle further deteriorated. In addition, the chances of developing a blood clot in your leg, then dying of the resultant pulmonary embolism (PE) went through the roof. (In PE, the clot in your leg breaks off and travels to the lungs where it gets stuck.)

In hospitals, death from MI has reduced from around 60 to about 9 per cent(ish). My figures here may be disputed, but this is a difficult area to pin down. Whatever the exact figures, things have got much better. And a great deal of this can be put down to earlier mobilisation following an MI, some of it due to drug treatment, some due to better control of electrical activity in the heart, some to PCI/ stenting, insertion of pacemakers and the use of implantable defibrillators. I feel that matters are now getting close to optimum in MI management.

What is certainly true is that if I had an MI, I would want to be whisked to the nearest big, shiny hospital where experienced doctors could do a PCI, thank you very much. Of course, I do not intend to have an MI as I am pretty certain that I know how to prevent it from happening, which reminds me of James Fixx, who stated that running would prevent him from having a heart attack. To quote the *New York Times*: 'James F. Fixx, who spurred the jogging craze with his best-selling books about running and preached the gospel that active people live longer, died of a heart attack Friday while on a solitary jog in Vermont. He was 52 years old.'[3]

Make of that, what you will. As a believer that exercise is indeed good for you, I will state that he would have died earlier if he had not taken up running. Other interpretations may be deemed valid.

STROKES

The other major disastrous event often caused by atherosclerosis is a stroke. As with heart attacks, there are variations on a theme. You will be glad to know there are only two basic types of stroke, but they do have a number of different causes.

The commonest type is an ischaemic stroke, ischaemia meaning lack of oxygen supply to a part of the body. This stroke is normally a two-step process. First, atherosclerotic plaques build-up in the carotid arteries in the neck, and then a blood clot forms over the plaque. Then, and this is where a stroke is different to an MI, the clot breaks off and travels up into the brain where it jams as the artery narrows. In turn this blocks the blood supply to an area of the brain, causing a cerebral infarct. Somewhat strangely, this is called a stroke and hardly ever a cerebral infarction (CI). You can also get infarcts deeper in the brain. These lacunar infarcts are usually smaller.

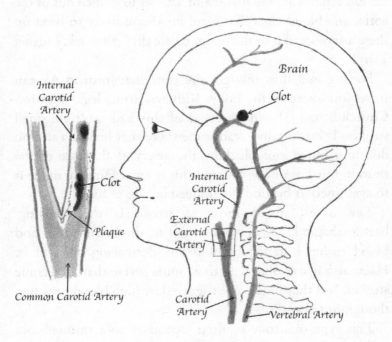

DIAGRAM 6

Another common cause of infarcts in the brain is AF. Here the upper chambers of the heart are fibrillating, i.e. not contracting in a controlled manner, somewhat like VF. However, because the contraction of the atria is much less critical to blood flow, people can live for many years with AF. In fact, there may not even be any symptoms.

However, AF is still a major health problem because, if the atria are fibrillating, the blood does not flow through smoothly and can form whirls and eddies, which makes it much more likely for clots to form. These can then break off, travel into the ventricles and then head for the heart. And because the carotid arteries are the first major arteries to branch out of the aorta, any blood clots that form in AF are likely to head up these arteries and into the brain, where they get stuck, causing a stroke.

Having said this, though, the clots that form in AF can travel anywhere in the body. Kidneys, arms, legs. Winston Churchill had AF, and because of this had multiple small strokes. I was certain I read somewhere that he lost a thumb due to a blood clot blocking the artery at the base of the thumb, but I am now not sure this is true. How he made it to age ninety is beyond the understanding of his GP. [4]

The other, major form of stroke is the bleeding, haemorrhagic kind. A blood vessel in the brain bursts and blood rushes into the brain tissue, destroying parts of it. Haemorrhagic strokes tend to be more severe than ischaemic strokes, and they tend to be triggered by high blood pressure, though not always.

This type of stroke is often secondary to a thinned and ballooned out area of the artery, an aneurysm. This weakened area is more likely to pop under pressure. If you have aneurysms in the arterial system at the base of the brain (the circle of Willis), they cause a subarachnoid haemorrhage. This is not quite the same as a stoke because the bleeding happens outside the brain, but it puts great pressure on the brain, forcing it down the spinal column and can cause severe damage – and death.

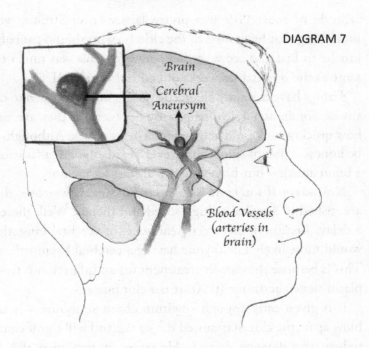

DIAGRAM 7

Brain

Cerebral
Aneursym

Blood Vessels
(arteries in
brain)

Finally, many strokes are defined as cryptogenic, which is a fancy way of saying, 'We don't know what caused it.' Doctors don't like saying that in any area of medicine, so pseudo-scientific terms have been developed to stop them admitting 'we simply haven't a clue'. Hence:

- Cryptogenic stroke = stroke of unknown cause
- Idiopathic pulmonary fibrosis = progressive lung damage of unknown cause
- Essential hypertension = high blood pressure of unknown cause

Anyway, back to strokes. When I was a fresh-faced young doctor, there was no effective treatment for strokes and the attitude of most GPs was pretty laissez-faire. Strokes were something that happened to the elderly, who should probably just lie in bed and see what happens. Yes, this was much the same as the original six weeks of bed rest for an MI.

Things have certainly changed. We are now supposed to call strokes 'brain attacks' to emphasise how serious they are, and how quickly we should act, as with a heart attack. Although, to be honest, I do not think I have ever heard anyone call a stroke a brain attack – but I am sure it will start happening.

Nowadays, if someone is suspected of having a stroke, they are rushed to hospital at high speed and then ... Well, there is a delay. Because the correct treatment for cerebral infarction would most likely kill anyone having a cerebral haemorrhage. This is because the correct treatment for an infarction is tissue plasminogen activator (tPA). It is a clot buster.

If it given early enough – within about six hours – it can blow apart the clot that caused the stroke and will significantly reduce the damage caused. However, if you give tPA to someone having a haemorrhagic stroke it will, instead, blow apart any clot that has formed to stop further bleeding into the brain, with drastic consequences.

Unfortunately, there is no way of knowing from the clinical signs if someone is having a cerebral infarct or a cerebral bleed. The only way to find out is with a brain scan, which means that you must try and get people suffering a stroke into a scanner as quickly as possible. If it is ischaemic, they get tPA. If it is a haemorrhage, they do not – they *must not*. About 80 per cent of strokes are ischaemic.

What I find fascinating is that if you have an MI, and the heart stops beating, irreversible brain damage occurs in about four to five minutes. If you have a stroke, and the blood stops flowing through a part of the brain, you can protect the rest of the brain if you give tPA within six hours. Maybe someone can explain this to me.

One drastic way to reduce the risk of ischaemic strokes is to look for large plaques in the carotid arteries and remove them surgically. You may have been offered a carotid artery scan as part of a health screen, which seem to be becoming increasingly popular. If you have greater than a certain amount of blockage, then a surgeon can open the artery and hook out most of the plaque. Sometimes they may put a stent in to keep the artery open. This can also be done after a stroke to stop another one happening in the future.

If you have AF, the treatment of choice is to take an anticoagulant to stop blood clots forming in the atria. The most commonly used anticoagulant in this case is warfarin (coumadin in the US). This is an extremely effective treatment and reduces the risk of stroke considerably. In a major study, warfarin reduced the risk of ischaemic stroke from 7.4 to 2.3 per cent per year.[5] For every hundred people that represents five fewer strokes per year, or fifty fewer over ten years. And that, my friends, is as good as any 'preventative' medicine ever gets. Of course, there are associated risks, such as an increased risk of bleeding, etc. But overall, in AF, I would advise warfarin asap.

In the last few years, newer, life-long anticoagulants have replaced warfarin. They are no more effective than warfarin, but they do not need to be monitored all the time – as with warfarin. You, your friends or relatives may have an (International Normalised Ratio) INR test every few weeks or so to check the dose of warfarin is correct. This is not needed with the newer drugs; however the newer drugs are about 80 times as expensive as warfarin. Kerchingggg!

At this point I think I have covered as much as you need to know about the underlying process of CVD. Essentially, it is a disease of the blood vessels themselves, consisting of thickened areas called atherosclerotic plaques. The final event is, usually, a blood clot forming on top of an already existing plaque.

The next questions are what causes the disease, and how to prevent it. However, before that, I think there is an equally pressing need to look in more detail at the factors currently considered to be the most important cause. Fat(s) and cholesterol in your diet, causing a raised blood cholesterol level, leading to atherosclerosis/atherosclerotic plaques.

CHAPTER 5

What are Fats?

The first thing to say here is that the terminology in this area is hopelessly confusing. I sometimes think there is a secret society out there, which has an evil plan to ensure that no one can understand anything about fats, cholesterol and the rest.

Just consider the word 'fat'. One can be fat, although no one can be called that any more. Fat can be removed from a steak, there are fat cells and you can call lots of fat cells clumped together fatty tissue. In addition, some people refer to triglycerides, which you may or may not have heard of, as fats. However, a triglyceride is also a lipoprotein, which is nothing like a fat at all. Having said all this, there is no such thing as a fat.

Confused? Well, I am not surprised. It took me some time to work out what anyone was talking about, so let's start with ...

FATTY ACIDS AND TRIGLYCERIDES

Whilst there is not such thing as a fat, there are fatty acids. These are generally what people are talking about they use the word fat. Fatty acids come in many different forms, and the terminology can seem quite daunting. For example, there is omega-3 fatty acid, which most people have heard of, usually as a part of super-healthy fish oils.

But what is it? Well, an omega-3 fatty acid is not a single entity. Omega 3s are available in a bewildering variety of forms. It is possible to have myristic omega-3 fatty acid or stearic omega-3 fatty acid. They can also be monounsaturated or polyunsaturated, with a -trans or -cis bond. Some could be considered healthy, others less so.

I know this may seem horribly off-putting, but the naming system is fairly simple to explain. Luckily fatty acids are also one of the simplest molecules in the human body. They consist of three elements. Carbon, oxygen and hydrogen. The backbone is a chain of carbon molecules that can vary in length from one to 80 carbon atoms, although anything over 20 is called 'long chain' and we can basically ignore anything over 30.

A fatty acid with 14 carbon atoms in the chain is called myristic acid, and a fatty acid with 16 carbon atoms is called palmitic acid because it was first found in palm oil in high concentrations. And when I tell you that napalm is made from palmitic acid, it does demonstrate that fatty acids contain a lot of energy.

The shortest and simplest fatty acid is acetic acid and still counts as a fatty acid, even though it has no chain of carbon atoms at all. Acetic acid can also be called vinegar (see diagram 8). Chemists do enjoy their world of total confusion.

DIAGRAM 8

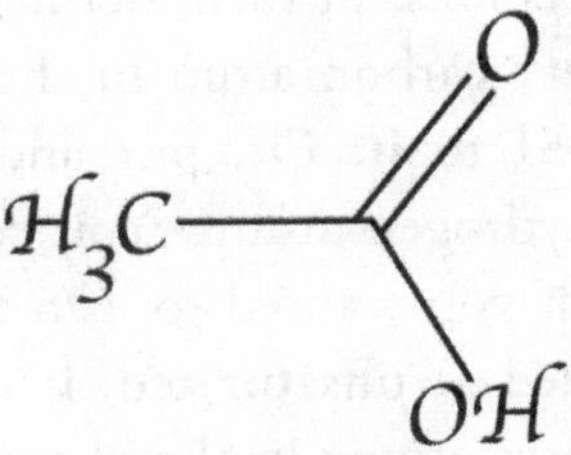

$$H_3C \diagdown \overset{\displaystyle O}{\underset{\displaystyle OH}{C}}$$

Acetic Acid

So when you visit the fish and chip shop, you could ask for 'Salt and saturated fatty acid on my chips please.' I don't imagine they'd have the faintest idea what you were talking about, though they might say, 'That'll raise your blood pressure and cholesterol, don't you know?'

Diagrams of fatty acids are normally presented as a chain of carbon atoms with hydrogen atoms attached along the chain. In Diagram 9 there are a total of 18 carbon atoms, which makes this one stearic acid. Incidentally, *stear* is the Greek for tallow, which is a rendered form of beef or mutton fat. And tallow, if you alter it a bit, can be used in jet engines as a biofuel and probably in any car with a diesel engine. At one time, beef tallow was also used by McDonald's to fry chips until they were told it was terribly unhealthy, and they should stop. Pity, because food fried in tallow is super delicious.

DIAGRAM 9

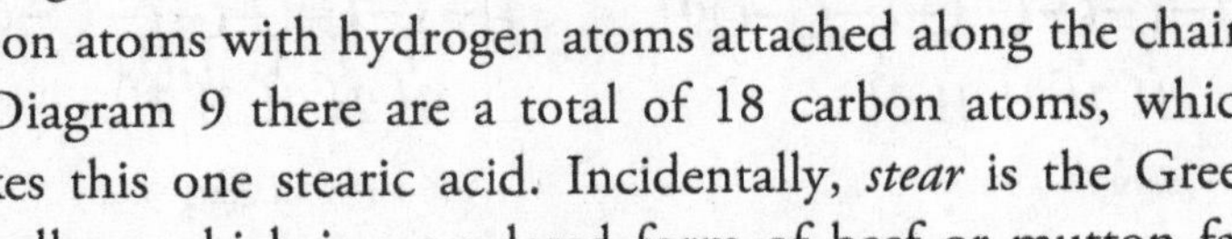

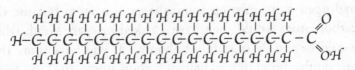

Stearic Acid, A saturated fatty acid

This stearic acid molecule is, in turn, defined as a saturated fatty acid because every carbon atom in the chain has two hydrogen atoms linked to it. Or, put another way, it is fully saturated with hydrogen atoms. You couldn't squeeze another one on even if you wanted to. On the other hand, if a fatty acid is defined as unsaturated, it is because there are (at least) two carbon atoms in the chain with only one hydrogen atom linked to them, in which case there is space for more hydrogen atoms. Or, let us say, it is unsaturated with hydrogen atoms.

DIAGRAM 10

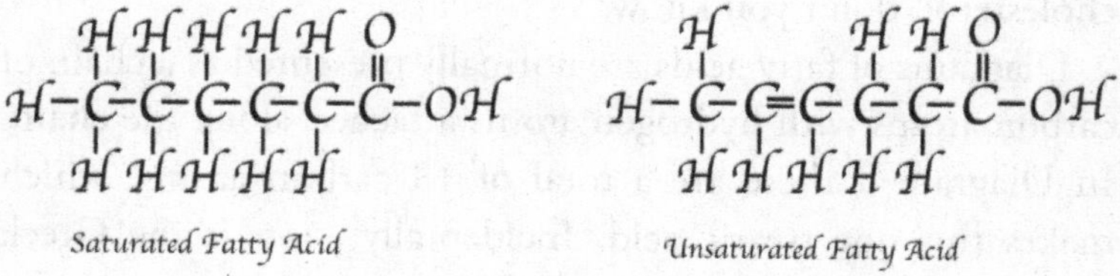

Saturated Fatty Acid   Unsaturated Fatty Acid

The relatively short, unsaturated fatty caproic acid in Diagram 10 is actually a *mono*unsaturated fatty acid because it has *two* carbon atoms, with no hydrogens attached. The reason for the prefix mono is that there is one double bond between two carbon atoms. Not that there is only one carbon atom with a single hydrogen attached. Please don't blame me for these naming systems. (Chemically, you could not have a single hydrogen atom missing from one carbon atom because that carbon atom would then have a naked or spare bond, which would be utterly unstable. Kaboom.) If you have more than one double bond in the chain of carbon atoms, the fatty acid is then referred to as a *poly*unsaturated fatty acid. The unsaturated fatty acid in the diagram below has three double bonds, and is missing six hydrogen atoms. This makes it polyunsaturated.

POLYUNSATURATED FATTY ACID

Polyunsaturated Fatty Acid

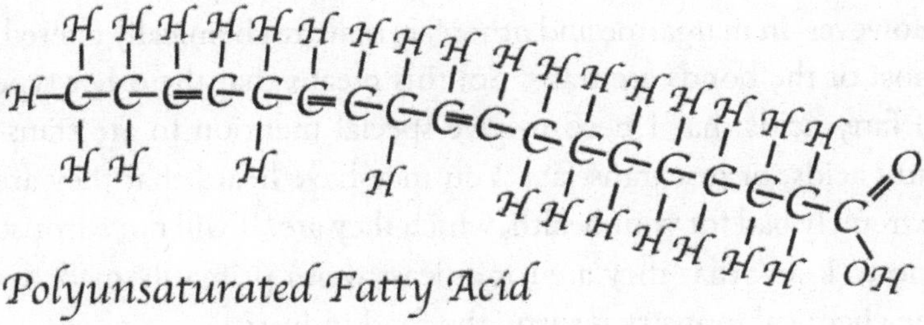

DIAGRAM 11

The other point of interest about this polyunsaturated fatty acid is that it is also an omega-3 unsaturated fatty acid. Fatty acids all have CH_3 at one end and COOH at the other, with a different number of CH_2s in the middle. The generic chemical formula is $CH_3(CH_2)_n COOH$. The COOH is the chemical part that makes all fatty acids mildly acidic.

The CH_3 end is called the omega end, and the COOH end is called the alpha end (as in from *alpha* to *omega*, the Greek for A to Z). However, weirdly, if a double bond is three from the omega end, it is called an omega-3 fatty acid, which means omega (minus) three, though if you want to show off then write 'ω-3 fatty acid'. In other words, you count backwards from the omega end of the fatty acid to get your omega number. I have never bothered to find out why it is done this way, it just is, probably to add yet another layer of confusion to a topic of almost maximum confusion. In fact, I suppose it is easier to count backwards towards the first double bond you can find.

There are two other points you need to know about fatty acids that are highly relevant to CVD. The first is that the double carbon bond in an unsaturated fatty acid can be in the -cis or -trans form. In nature, virtually every bond is cis. However, in margarine and other fats that are chemically altered, most of the bonds are trans. So, this means that the other type of fatty acids that I need to give special mention to are trans-fatty acids, or just trans-fats. You may have heard that they are extremely bad for your health, which they are. It will not surprise you to know that they are (or at least were) primarily made by the chemical industry – sorry, the food industry.

Why are they called trans? Well, you can have two types of bond in an unsaturated fatty acid. The first is a -cis bond, where both hydrogens are missing from the same side (yes, any chemist reading that will no doubt choke on their morning Oreo). On the other hand, a trans-fat is where the hydrogen atoms are missing from different sides.

DIAGRAM 12

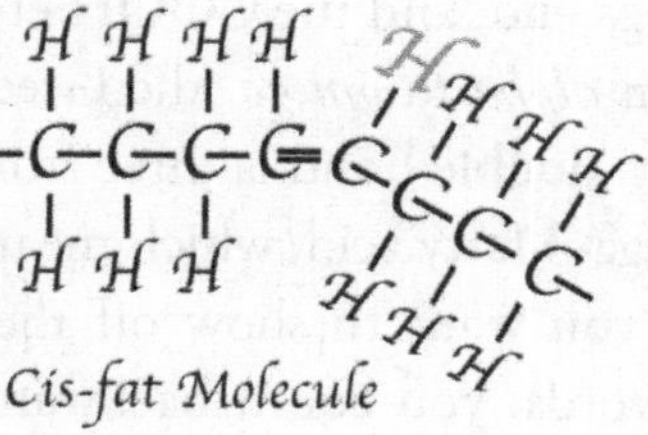

Cis-fat Molecule 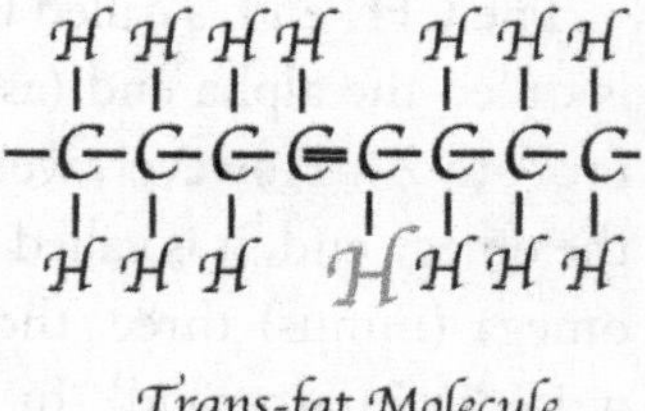   Trans-fat Molecule

As you can see from this highly oversimplified molecule, a cis-fatty acid is bent in the middle. A trans-fatty acid is straight. For the food industry, this very slight difference becomes highly important. Because ... sorry, aaarrrggghhh, when I started writing about fatty acids I thought it would take a couple of pages. As with almost anything it ends up more complicated than you thought. Oh well, onwards and upwards.

Anyway, most saturated fatty acids, especially the longer ones, are solid at room temperature (clearly, acetic acid is not) because they tend to be straight. Unsaturated fatty acids, at least those with -cis bonds, can bend and wobble in the middle and will not pack together so tightly, which makes them liquid at room temperature. At this point they are not called fats, they are oils. Yes, an oil is just a liquid fat or, to be more accurate, liquid fatty acids.

Therefore, if you want a healthy polyunsaturated substance to put on your toast you have a problem. Whilst you can dip bread into olive oil at fancy restaurants, you cannot really spread oil, it makes a hell of a mess and drips all over your clothes. If you want to create semi-solid poly-unsaturated fatty acids, you need to convert the bonds from cis to trans. Then they won't bend in the middle, can be packed together more tightly and will be solid at room temperature. Clear?

Twisting, superheating and mangling polyunsaturated fats in this way results in that super-healthy substance called margarine. You may remember margarine. Indeed, I think it is now only possible *to remember* it because it seems that it no longer exists. It was pointed out to me recently that margarine has disappeared, like the Cheshire Cat, leaving only a smile. It cannot be found on the shelves of supermarkets. What we have instead are low-fat spreads. And last time I walked round Sainsbury's, there was no margarine, only new, improved, low-fat spreads. How strange.

What is the difference between a low-fat spread and margarine? I had a quick look on Google, and this was what I came across from some PR company blub. 'Choose low-fat and reduced-fat spreads and oils such as rapeseed or olive oil (monounsaturated) instead of hard margarine, lard or butter. To have a low level of saturated fat, which is very important for your heart, you need to limit butter to once a week ... Choose lower fat options.' And that's distinctly weird because low-fat spreads are still made, almost exclusively, from fatty acids, chemically mangled or not. So, a low-fat spread has the same amount of fat in it as butter – see terminology transforming in front of our eyes.

Margarine was, at one point, advertised as super-healthy because it was high in polyunsaturated fatty acids rather than those deadly, saturated fatty acids. However, the polyunsaturated fatty acids in margarine were primarily trans-fats, which were later found to be uniquely bad for health. So bad that they now been banned in many countries. The consequence of this is that margarine has transformed from being uniquely healthy to uniquely unhealthy. In a strange coincidence, margarine has magically disappeared from supermarket shelves to be replaced by 'low-fat' spreads, i.e. 'low fat' to anyone in an advertising agency. Oh well, language is a funny old thing, is it not? George Orwell would, no doubt, be spinning in his grave. 'Eat low-fat fat instead of high-fat fat.' You know it makes perfect sense. That thudding noise in the background is a chemist beating his head repeatedly against the wall.

One thing that I find intriguing, but have not yet found an answer to, is the following question. How have the manufacturers of these new 'high-fat low-fat' (HFLF) spreads managed to make them solid at room temperature without changing the bonds from cis to trans? I have looked at the website of one leading manufacturer in some detail, and it claims that there are no longer any trans-fats or partially hydrogenated fats in in its product, although I know that there were in the past. If this is true, their product should be an oil, but it is not. I think they have hydrogenated the plant sterols instead – if, indeed, that is possible. Their explanations how they now make polyunsaturated fats solid are totally ... well, let's be kind, beyond my understanding.

Of course, there is a delicious irony to the entire trans-fat saga, which would be funny if it had not resulted in so many premature deaths. We now know that trans-fats are one of *the* unhealthiest things you can put in your mouth. To quote *Wikipedia*: 'Trans-fats, or trans-unsaturated fatty acids, trans-fatty acids, are a type of unsaturated fat that occur in small amounts in nature, but became widely produced industrially from vegetable fats for use in margarine, snack food, packaged baked goods and frying fast food starting in the 1950s. Trans-fat has been shown to consistently be associated, in an intake-dependent way, with increased risk of coronary artery disease, a leading cause of death in Western nations.'

However, at one time, such were the unquestioned benefits of polyunsaturated fatty acids, which included trans-fats, that in the 1980s there was a mass movement to ban McDonald's from using beef tallow to fry chips, as this was seen as terribly unhealthy. McDonald's always get it in the neck from everyone.

Under extreme pressure, McDonald's and many other restaurants were forced to give up beef tallow and started frying in the newer 'super-healthy trans-fats'. This was primarily due to a campaign run by an organisation called the Centre for Science in the Public Interest (CSPI). The CSPI is now the most active critic of trans-fats. The whole sorry saga of replacing super-healthy, saturated fatty acids with deadly trans-fats is well covered by an article entitled 'The Tragic Legacy of Centre for Science in the Public Interest (CSPI)'.[1]

Anyway, where was I? Oh yes, there is no such thing as fat. There are fatty acids, which can be of different lengths, and they can be fully saturated or unsaturated. They can have a -cis or -trans double bond, and if the double bond is three along from the omega end, they are called omega-3 fatty acids, which you find in fish oil. If the double bond is six along from the omega end they are called omega-6 fatty acids, etc.

Apart from trans-fats, they are all perfectly healthy, and there is no strong evidence that any are better or worse for you. Certain animal-sourced omega-3s may have specific benefits, but I wouldn't go overboard about them.

The final thing that you need to know about fatty acids is that they rarely travel alone in nature. They are normally bundled together in threes. To be more accurate, three fatty acids are attached to a glycerol molecule and create a triglyceride. A triglyceride is what's found in fat cells and is sometimes called fat, as in 'triglycerides are fats'.

CHAPTER 6

Triglycerides

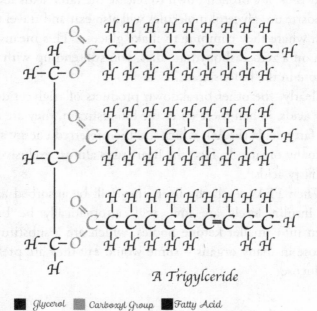

A Trigylceride

■ *Glycerol*   ■ *Carboxyl Group*   ■ *Fatty Acid*

DIAGRAM 13

In this chemical diagram of a triglyceride, we have two saturated fatty acids at the top of the triglyceride and one monounsaturated fatty acid at the bottom with a -cis bond. You can have any combination of fatty acids in a triglyceride. One saturated and two monounsaturated, all monounsaturated, all polyunsaturated, etc.

There are a few other things you need to know about triglycerides. Because the acidic end 'COOH' is now bound to glycerol, a triglyceride is not acidic, it is Ph neutral, neither acid nor alkali. Of additional interest, the backbone of a triglyceride is a glycerol molecule, and each glycerol molecule is one half of a glucose molecule. When triglycerides, stored in fat cells, are broken down to release the fatty acids into the bloodstream, glycerol molecules will also exit and travel to the liver, where they combine to make glucose. This means that, even on a zero-carbohydrate diet, you still end up with some glucose in the bloodstream.

Clearly, the other breakdown products of triglycerides are fatty acids. When these enter the bloodstream, they are called free fatty acids (FFAs), which are the preferred energy source for many organs. In fact, the heart runs almost exclusively on free fatty acids.[1]

When FFAs reach the liver, they will be absorbed and, if the insulin levels are low, will automatically be broken down into smaller ketone bodies, which are a substitute for glucose in many organs – some would say they are preferred to glucose.

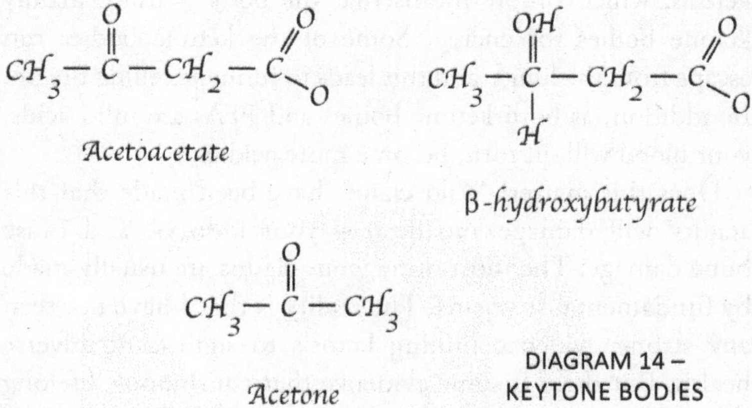

$$CH_3 - \overset{\overset{O}{\|}}{C} - CH_2 - \overset{\overset{O}{\|}}{C} \diagdown_O \qquad CH_3 - \overset{\overset{OH}{\|}}{\underset{\underset{H}{|}}{C}} - CH_2 - \overset{\overset{O}{\|}}{C} \diagdown_O$$

Acetoacetate

β-hydroxybutyrate

$$CH_3 - \overset{\overset{O}{\|}}{C} - CH_3$$

Acetone

**DIAGRAM 14 –
KEYTONE BODIES**

When blood glucose levels are low, the brain receives 60–70 per cent of the energy it needs from ketone bodies. The heart will also use ketone bodies, alongside FFAs, for energy rather than glucose, as do many other organs.

This preference for ketone bodies over glucose should not really be surprising. The body can store, literally, millions of calories as triglycerides/fatty acids, and only around 1,500 calories as glucose/glycogen. Ergo, the body must be perfectly adapted to use fatty acids and ketone bodies for energy or it could not function. Bears in hibernation, for example, have no choice but to live off fat stores for up to six months, and it does them no harm, although they get a bit grumpy when they wake up.

You do not need to get into such an extreme metabolic state as hibernation before your body stops using glucose as the primary energy source. After fasting for a day, your glucose/glycogen stores will be running dry. Then your metabolism happily switches over, at which point you enter the state of ketosis, which simply means that the body is using mainly ketone bodies for energy. Some of the ketone bodies can escape from the lungs, and this leads to funny-smelling breath. In addition, as both ketone bodies and FFAs are mild acids, your blood will, in turn, become more acidic.

Does this matter? Wild claims have been made that this acidity will damage and destroy your kidneys, and cause bone damage. The most outrageous claims are usually made by fundamentalist vegans. The reality is that I have not seen any strong evidence linking ketosis to significant adverse health. But there is some evidence that continuous, lifelong ketosis may create problems in a few individuals.[2] On the other hand, people with resistant epilepsy have found that ketosis will often 'cure' their disease. This is well accepted and non-contentious. But most people are never going to remain entirely carbohydrate-restricted year after year, and I would not recommend this unless you have intractable epilepsy. There are some who do, and those who follow the anti-carb 'paleo' diet would have us all ruthlessly expunge carbohydrates from our diet and eat virtually nothing but animal products.

Why, oh why, do people have to go to such extremes? I am fully on board with eating natural foods and drastically cutting down on the carbs, especially if you have diabetes. But you don't need to go completely bonkers. Our ancestors ate fruit and nuts, and whatever vegetables they could find. We are not designed to be carb-free, nor should we try to be.

Another problem is that people mix up ketosis and ketoacidosis. They sound similar, but they are not the same. One is perfectly healthy, one deadly. Ketosis occurs in anyone who doesn't eat for a day. Ketoacidosis will only occur if you have type 1 diabetes, the type of diabetes when the body cannot produce insulin.

Insulin, amongst other things, keeps triglycerides trapped in fat cells. This is because insulin is primarily an energy-storage hormone, and one of its roles is to ensure that fatty acids are stored, not released. If the insulin level drops too low, and stays low, triglycerides break down into FFAs and then flood out into the bloodstream. When they reach the liver, they are automatically converted to ketone bodies, and this unstoppable avalanche will turn the blood more and more acidic until you enter a keto-acidotic coma. And you die.

Ketoacidosis, ketosis. Do not get these very similar terms confused. But if you do, you will be in good company, alongside 90 per cent of medics who hear 'keto'... then run, screaming in terror. Straight to the nearest McDonald's.

Anyway, at this point, I hope that you have a better handle on what fatty acids are, and how they fit into the human metabolism, and how to understand the terminology surrounding fatty acids, etc. Unfortunately, there is one further area of potential confusion that I need to clarify, which is the word lipid. You may have heard of blood lipids or lipid levels. Are they the same as fats/fatty acids?

To quote Medicine.net on lipids: 'Lipids: Another word for "fats". Lipids can be more formally defined as substances such as a fat, oil or wax that dissolves in alcohol but not in water. Lipids contain carbon, hydrogen and oxygen but have far less oxygen proportionally than carbohydrates.'

Yes, fats can be called lipids and lipids are fats. The two words are interchangeable. Just to make things clear, here is my little ready reckoner:

Fatty acid = fat
Triglyceride = fat
Lipid = fat
Fat = lipid

Clear? The unfortunate fact is that, in this area, people interchange terminology all the time. This does not make it easy to follow what they are talking about. In fact, I often wonder if they have any idea themselves. At least now, I hope, you have a good grasp of this whole area.

CHAPTER 7

What is Cholesterol?

Cholesterol, the harbinger of death. Or is it? I have seen cholesterol defined as many different things: a lipid, a fat, a sterol, an alcohol and an organic compound belonging to the steroid family. Well, the more you learn, the more confused you get. You would think someone, somewhere, could decide what it is. In fact, it would be nice if they could decide what anything is. Failing that, at least we could agree on what to call it.

Chemically, at least, it is very clear what cholesterol is. It has the chemical formula $C_{27}H_{46}O$. Yes, just like fats and sugars it is entirely made from oxygen, hydrogen and carbon atoms. Anyone would think there is a theme emerging here. The chemical diagram looks like this:

DIAGRAM 15

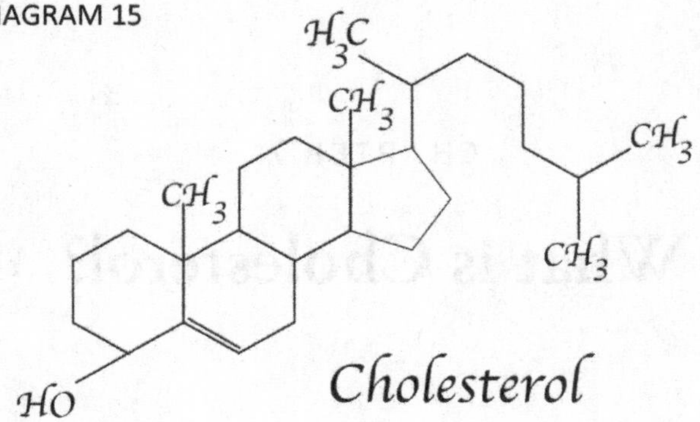

Cholesterol

Now, close your eyes for a moment and think about the structure of a fatty acid. Now open them and look at the chemical structure of cholesterol. See, they are the same – are they not? Well, here is what the National Institutes of Health has to say: 'Cholesterol is a waxy, fat-like substance that's found in all cells of the body.' Fat-like? Well, I suppose it has carbon, hydrogen and oxygen molecules in it. Otherwise?

Despite this, I certainly agree with the last bit of their statement. Cholesterol *is* found in all cells of the body. Indeed, if all the cells of your body did not contain lots of cholesterol, you would be dead. To quote from Chris Masterjohn: 'Cholesterol is found in every cell of your body. It is especially abundant in the membranes of these cells, where it helps maintain the integrity of these membranes, and plays a role in facilitating cell signalling – meaning the ability of your cells to communicate with each other so you function as a human, rather than a pile of cells ... Without cholesterol, cell membranes would be too fluid, not firm enough, and too permeable to some molecules. In other words, it keeps the membrane from turning to mush.'[1]

If you remember biology from your school days, animals have cells with cell membranes surrounding them. On the other hand, plants have cell walls, which are far more rigid and unbending. So, instead of having vast amounts of cholesterol in their cell walls, plants have plant stanols/sterols, which do much the same thing for plant cells as cholesterol does for animal cells.

And that explains why cholesterol, apart from being a lipid, a fat, an alcohol and a steroid is also called a stanol, or a sterol. As they have the same basic function in cells, sterols and cholesterol are pretty similar. You can now play spot the difference between cholesterol and a sterol.

DIAGRAM 16

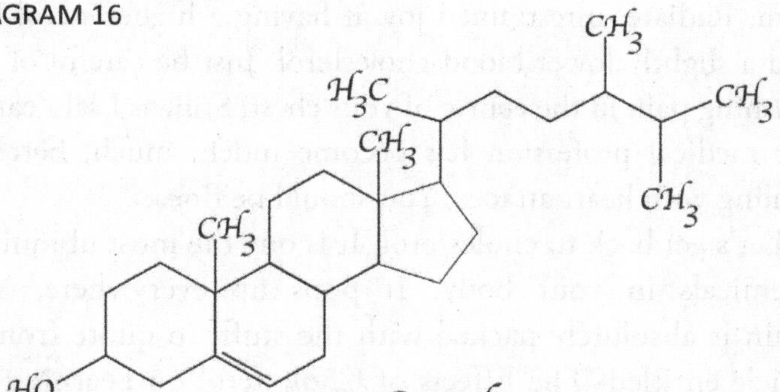

Sterol

You may have heard of plant sterols before, mainly because they are artificially stuck into Benecol and other super-healthy, low-fat spreads. Food manufacturers do this because sterols/stanols 'lower blood cholesterol'. Whoopee.

But is it a good idea to stick plant sterols into humans, when we are physiologically designed to use cholesterol? It seems unlikely. What we have here is the same type of thinking that led to the replacement of saturated fats with trans-fats. To quote the *Journal of Biological Sciences*: 'It is widely accepted that cholesterol lowering is healthful per se. We challenge this view, with particular reference to plant sterols. Cholesterol lowering should not be an end in itself. The objective must be to reduce health outcomes, such as incidence of Coronary Heart Disease (CHD). We hypothesised that plant sterols may lower cholesterol, but not CHD. *We found the outcome on CHD in fact to be detrimental.*'[2]

In short, if you eat plant sterols, cholesterol levels *will* go down but mortality goes up. This effect is not massive, but it has been found consistently, in many different studies. So, enjoy your 'plant-sterol-enhanced-low-fat-spreads', yum, yum. Radiate unrestrained joy at having a higher sterol level and a slightly lower blood cholesterol. Just be careful of that crushing pain in the centre of your chest. Still, as I said earlier, the medical profession has become much, much, better at dealing with heart attacks. You should be fine.

Let's get back to cholesterol. It is one the most ubiquitous chemicals in your body. It pops up everywhere. Your brain is absolutely packed with the stuff, to quote from an article entitled 'The Effects of Cholesterol on Learning and Memory': 'Cholesterol is ubiquitous in the central nervous system (CNS) and vital to normal brain function including signalling, synaptic plasticity, and learning and memory. Cholesterol is so important to brain function that it is generated independently of cholesterol metabolism in the rest of the body and is sequestered from the body by the blood brain barrier (BBB).'[3]

To explain that last bit. The brain must manufacture its own cholesterol. It needs to do this because – as far as I can establish, which is more difficult than you might imagine –

cholesterol cannot get into the brain from the bloodstream. It is blocked by the BBB.

A few other key points emerge from that short quote. First, cholesterol is essential for the formation of synapses, and the creation of new synapses is the way that memories are created and stored. Second, cholesterol is critical for the health of neurones, as it makes up most of the myelin sheath. This protective sheath surrounds and nurtures neurones, and allows them to function.

To further emphasise the need for cholesterol in the brain, there is a rare disease called Smith-Lemli-Opitz Syndrome (SLOS). Those born with SLOS have a very low cholesterol level, due to an inborn error of cholesterol synthesis. They also have a wide spectrum of defects, including microcephaly (a very small brain). This is because their neurones cannot develop properly, due to a lack of cholesterol.

Yes, let us prescribe statins to children, with still-developing brains, and see what happens ... let me guess. I suspect not many of them will get to university, although several may make it into government. And they might even be prime minister or president.

Apart from being synthesised within the brain, where does cholesterol come from? Well, as it is found in all animal cells, you will consume cholesterol if you eat almost any part of any animal. The highest concentration is found in sea food and egg yolks. The egg yolk is, as we all know, what the bird embryo uses to feed on and grow. The reason why there is a hell of a lot of cholesterol in egg yolks is because it takes a hell of a lot of cholesterol to construct a healthy bird.

Having said this, you only get a small amount of your cholesterol from your diet. Most of the cholesterol you need is made in the liver. Cholesterol synthesis is a very complex 37-step process, which I am not going to delve into in any detail. However, one important step is when the chemical compound 3-hydroxy-3-methylglutaryl CoA (HMG-CoA) is converted to mevalonate by the enzyme HMG-CoA reductase.

The only reason I added this bit of rather off-putting biochemistry is that, if you block HMG-CoA reductase, then you block cholesterol production. The reason for mentioning this is because statins are HMG-CoA reductase inhibitors. That is how they work. Ah, the wonders of medical science. The body is desperately trying to make cholesterol to ensure perfect health and wellbeing, and we blithely throw a spanner into a complex 37-step process, one that is essential for human existence. Splendid idea, chaps.

Anyway, apart from ensuring that the brain, the neurones and all cells in the body develop and function properly, what else does cholesterol do? Well, once nature finds a good chemical, it tends to adapt it in various ways to do all sorts of different things, and cholesterol is no exception. It is the backbone for many hormones. They include:

- Aldosterone
- Cortisol
- Oestrogens
- Progesterone
- Testosterone and DHEA
- Vitamin D (I've included this as a steroid hormone. It is usually described as a vitamin but I think that is simply wrong. It has the same basic chemical structure as many other hormones, and it acts like a hormone.)

There is a delicious irony at this point because vitamin D is increasingly recognised as being beneficial for heart health, and where do we get most of our vitamin D from? Well, I am glad you asked. It is synthesised in the skin, from cholesterol, by the action of sunlight. Yes, the terrible, deadly substance that must be lowered forms the essential building block for a vital hormone.

At this point I shall interrupt this tightly structured narrative to take you on a couple of detours. In another of those intriguing twists in science, there are some researchers who believe that the beneficial effect of statins do not result from their cholesterol-lowering action, but because they are vitamin D analogues. By which I mean they have actions you would normally associate with vitamin D.

Superficially, this may sound highly unlikely. However, if you delve more deeply into the science, this idea is not as crazy as it may seem. Most drugs achieve their effects in the body by closely mimicking things they are either trying to stimulate or block. Or, to put this another way, if you want to stop, say, an enzyme functioning, you lob a chemical at it, one that looks pretty much like the chemical that the enzyme was designed to convert into something else in the first place.

So, if an enzyme is trying to turn chemical A into chemical B – or bond chemical A to B – and you want to prevent this happening, you throw chemical A^1 at it. Chemical A^1 can be almost identical to A, apart from one small tweak. There may be extra hydrogen attached, or a different side chain of some sort. The alien chemical A^1 then sits within the active site of the enzyme and does not move. The enzyme is now blocked, to a greater or lesser extent.

I think I probably need to provide a bit more information on enzymes at this point. They are the most amazing machines. They are, just to give one important example (important to me, anyway), responsible for converting sugar into alcohol, which you may think of as a good or a bad thing. I think it is a good thing.

There are about 75,000 enzymes inside your body, and without them almost every biochemical process would grind to a complete halt. How best to think of them? Lock and key ... maybe. I struggle to think of a perfect analogy and I don't want to get dragged into trying to explain stereoisomers or racemic mixes.

Keeping this as simple as possible, enzymes either break molecules apart or join them together. Whichever way round, if you want the correct reaction to occur, you need one molecule to be held in a specific position in order that it can more easily line up with another molecule. Once both molecules are correctly aligned, the desired chemical reactions will take place.

If you relied on chance to get the precise lining up to occur, that is, two molecules bumping into each other, in exactly the correct alignment, you could wait a long, long time for anything to happen. However, when an enzyme 'holds' one molecule in its active site (the bit the molecule fits into), the next molecule can slot alongside and, hey presto, the reaction occurs. The newly created molecule floats away and the enzyme is ready to go again.

It has been estimated that some chemical reactions, if you just waited for them to happen by chance, would take the entire lifespan of the universe to occur. But add an enzyme and the reaction can take place in less than one second. To look at this in another time dimension, there are enzymes in the body that are capable of 'catalysing' specific chemical reactions one million times per second. And if that doesn't boggle your mind, nothing will. I can't think of anything happening one million times a second; it is beyond my comprehension.

In case you are interested, the enzymes working this fast are carbonic anhydrases, which 'catalyse' the conversion of carbon dioxide and water into bicarbonate and protons (or vice versa). In humans, this process maintains the acid-base balance in your cells, and helps to transport carbon dioxide out of tissues, which is vital. And, just to repeat, it can do this one million times a second. So, if anyone says you are lazy, tell them that – even if it is looks as if you are sitting there doing nothing – you are inter-converting carbon dioxide and bicarbonate quicker than ...

All of which means that, if you want to stop a chemical reaction dead in its tracks, find another molecule that will sit passively in the active site of an important enzyme. This will block its ability to catalyse reactions, and that will be that. Penicillin, for example, is an irreversible enzyme inhibitor that stops bacteria from synthesising a vital constituent of cell walls, so the bacteria simply burst open and die – until they develop resistance.

Whilst some molecules can act as irreversible blockers, others compete for the active site with the original chemical, so they slow down – rather than stop – reactions. Many enzyme blockers are themselves broken down and removed, which means that their actions are temporary. Statins are competitive inhibitors of the enzyme HMG-CoA, and they are broken down and cleared away over a couple of days or so.

Now, attempting to pull these strands together, if you

find a substance that is going to stop cholesterol from being synthesised, it will usually have certain critical similarities to cholesterol. This will enable it to get stuck in the enzyme's active site, blocking the reaction. Furthermore, this means that structurally statins must have some cholesterol-like qualities or else they could not jam up the enzyme HMG-CoA. By extension, this means they may also have vitamin D-like qualities, as vitamin D is synthesised from cholesterol. Ergo, it is possible that statins do have vitamin D-like effects throughout the body, which means that any benefits they provide could be due to action as D analogues.

I am not saying this is true, but I am trying to give you some idea of the mind-boggling complexity of human physiology. Inside us everything is connected to everything else, in ways that may seem almost impossible at first sight.

And if you think it is a wild stretch to believe that cholesterol and vitamin D are closely related. Here are the chemical diagrams for cholesterol and vitamin D.

DIAGRAM 17

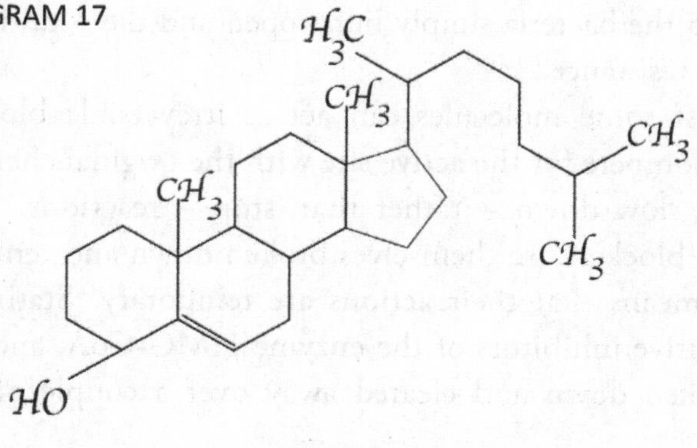

CHOLESTEROL

DIAGRAM 17

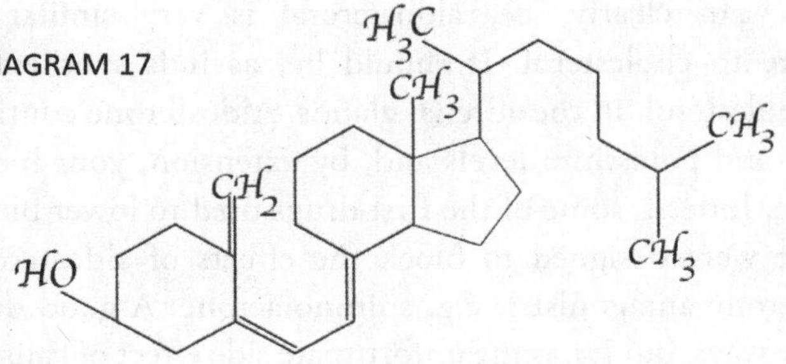

VITAMIN D

Looking at this diagram, you can also deduce that our bodies certainly like to conserve energy. After expending a great deal of effort synthesising cholesterol, with its complex hydrocarbon rings, etc., it then goes on to use cholesterol as the building block for all sorts of other things. And why not? This is evolution in action; small changes to a basic structure to achieve many different benefits.

Here, to give you another example of what cholesterol can turn into, is a hormone called aldosterone, which you have probably never heard of.

DIAGRAM 18

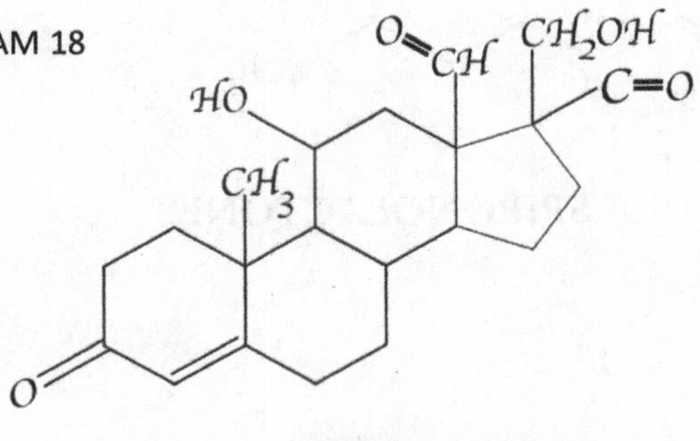

ALDOSTERONE

As you can clearly see, aldosterone is very similar in structure to cholesterol. It should be, as it is synthesised from cholesterol, in the adrenal glands. Aldosterone controls sodium and potassium levels and, by extension, your blood pressure. Indeed, some of the first drugs used to lower blood pressure were designed to block the effects of aldosterone (aldosterone antagonists), e.g. spironolactone. A good drug in many ways, but it has the unfortunate side effect of causing breast tissue growth in men (gynaecomastia). This is not entirely surprising because, in a certain light, spironolactone can look rather like oestrogen, the female sex hormone that stimulates breast growth in women.

DIAGRAM 19

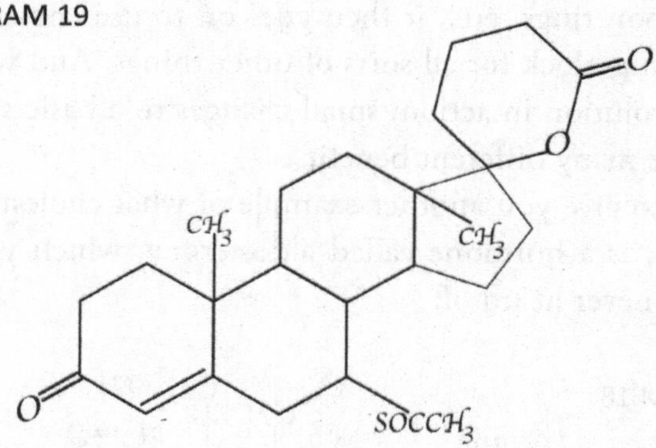

SPIRONOLACTONE

DIAGRAM 20

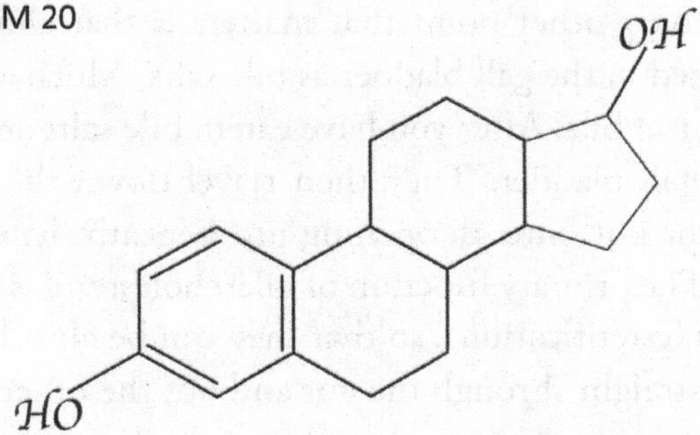

OESTROGEN

Oestrogen, in turn, is known to raise blood pressure, possibly because it has aldosterone-like effects. Statins, on the other hand, can lower blood pressure by as much, if not more, than many anti-hypertensives (blood pressure lowering drugs). Perhaps statins also block the effects of aldosterone and oestrogen?

Okay, enough of that. I must admit that I find this stuff endlessly fascinating, although when I was learning about it at medical school it seemed anything but. I had to beat my head against the desk repeatedly to stay awake. Perhaps the way this stuff was taught did not connect with my brain.

Anyway, I hope it is now clear that statins may be a form of vitamin D analogue and may have a beneficial effect on CVD by pretending to be vitamin D, and this isn't a completely ridiculous idea. That does not, of course, make the hypothesis correct. However, it does help to set the scene for later on when I will look more closely at the idea that, whilst statins do have some benefits on CVD, this has nothing whatsoever to do with their effect on lowering cholesterol levels.

Getting back to the functions of cholesterol in the body, I think the only other point that matters is that cholesterol is concentrated in the gall bladder as bile salts, which are the key constituent of bile. After you have eaten, bile salts are excreted from the gall bladder. They then travel down the bile duct and into the gut, into an opening just beneath the exit of the stomach. The primary function of bile/cholesterol is to bind to fatty acids (esterification), so that they can be absorbed rather than pass straight through the gut and out the other end.

Gallstones can obstruct the release of bile salts/cholesterol by blocking the bile duct. So, you can get a pain after eating a fatty meal as the gall bladder goes into a spasm as it tries to force bile past the obstruction. You may also get somewhat horrible bowel motions as they will be full of undigested fat, a symptom known as steatorrhea (bulky, offensive, fatty stools). Gallstones are primary made of crystallised cholesterol.

Most of the cholesterol within bile salts is reabsorbed and recycled by the liver. Therefore, one way to lower the cholesterol levels is to give drugs that bind to the bile salts/cholesterol, which will then be excreted in your stools. Medications that did this, such as cholestyramine, were used in the PS (pre-statin) era. They were reasonably effective at lowering cholesterol levels but were horrible to take and caused some rather smelly, adverse effects, along with stomach cramps. In addition, in clinical trials, they had zero benefit on mortality. The updated version of cholestyramine is called ezetimibe, and some people are still prescribed this to lower blood cholesterol – for reasons beyond the understanding of man, or indeed, woman.

CHAPTER 8

What is Your Blood Cholesterol Level?

As with fats, we have an immediate problem with terminology. The first issue is that you have no cholesterol floating free in your bloodstream, so it is impossible to have a blood cholesterol level. Scientifically, it cannot and does not exist. But the concept of a high cholesterol level has become so firmly concreted into the public consciousness that I am rather stuck with using it. (I am also going to use the generic term 'lipid' from now on, except when this is not possible.)

Incidentally, the reason why cholesterol does not float about in the bloodstream is that it does not dissolve in water – thus blood. It shares this problem with lipids, such as triglycerides. Therefore the only way you can transport cholesterol and triglycerides around is to pack them into lipoproteins – a lipid/protein sphere.

Lipoproteins come in various sizes and do different jobs. Here is a list, from the smallest to biggest:

HDL – High-density lipoprotein (often called 'good' cholesterol)

LDL – Low-density lipoprotein (often called 'bad' cholesterol)

IDL – Intermediate-density lipoprotein (usually not talked about in polite company)

VLDL – Very low-density lipoprotein (confusingly, usually called a triglyceride)

Chylomicron – although it's a lipoprotein it is not called a lipoprotein

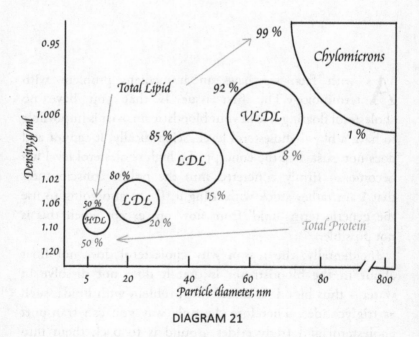

DIAGRAM 21

As you can see from the diagram, a chylomicron is enormous compared to HDL. Jupiter v Mercury. It is almost entirely made up of triglycerides, which means that 99 per cent of a chylomicron is lipid, the other 1 per cent is protein. On the other hand, HDL is 50 per cent lipid and 50 cent protein.

The other key fact about lipoproteins is that they have different, and complex, proteins stuck to the outside, which allow them to be identified by receptors on most cells throughout the body; they then latch onto them, lock and key. The attached proteins are apolipoproteins.

The main identifier protein on a chylomicron is apolipoprotein B-48 (Apo B-48). The main identifier protein on LDL is apolipoprotein B-100 (Apo B-100). You may have come across people offering to measure your Apo B-100 level, rather than your cholesterol level, in which case keep your bank account details well away from them and run like the wind.

Chylomicrons are the simplest of the lipoproteins to explain. They are created in the gut after eating a meal that contains fat/lipid. They then leave the gut and travel straight into the bloodstream, via a special vessel called the thoracic duct. Unlike all other foodstuffs, they do not go straight from the gut to the liver. They bypass it completely. Indeed, after eating a high fat/lipid meal, the blood can turn white due to the very high concentration of chylomicrons floating about. Despite this, no one thinks chylomicrons have any association with CVD. At least, I have never seen this proposed by anyone, anywhere. Maybe I need to look harder.

Basically, chylomicrons start life as bloated lipid spheres in the gut. They are released directly into the circulation, lock onto B-48 receptors on fat cells, their triglycerides are unloaded and they shrink right down until they become a chylomicron remnant. At which point this shrivelled-up remnant is absorbed into the liver where it is broken down, and the resulting products are used to construct other things.

When it comes to VLDLs, matters get a little bit more complicated. Unlike chylomicrons, VLDLs are constructed within the liver, not the gut. They too contain triglyceride, but they have a far higher percentage of cholesterol. The basic function of a VLDL is to transport newly synthesised triglycerides and cholesterol out of the liver, to be taken up and used in other cells and organs around the body. Just to keep you utterly confused, it has been decreed that VLDLs are also called triglycerides. If you have been told you have a high triglyceride level, you have a high VLDL level.

Like chylomicrons, VLDLs lose triglyceride and shrivel down in size to become IDLs. As they get even smaller, they transform into an LDL. And, because they lose triglyceride as they shrink, the proportion of cholesterol within LDL is higher than in a VLDL. In the end, up to 50 per cent of an LDL can be made up of cholesterol. Most of the LDLs do nothing further, and are simply absorbed back into the liver and broken down.

The alternative fate of LDL is to latch onto an LDL receptor on another cell in the body, before being pulled out of the bloodstream. Most cells can manufacture their own cholesterol, but they prefer to get it from LDL. When a cell needs extra cholesterol, it manufactures an LDL receptor and then sticks it out through the cell membrane to grab hold of a passing LDL molecule and pull it in. Once inside the cell, the LDL + receptor complex is broken down, and the cholesterol and triglyceride are used for various functions. The only exception to this is what happens in the brain. As touched on earlier, LDL cannot pass through the BBB, so the brain needs to synthesise its own cholesterol.

But what about HDLs, the fabled 'good' cholesterol? It is

still unclear, at least it remains unclear to me, exactly where it comes from. Some from the liver, some from the guts and some of from outer space, for all I can make of it. Wherever it comes from, though, it is constantly reforming and changing its structure all the time, shedding and transferring various apolipoproteins.

Currently, it has been decreed that HDL, a.k.a. 'good' cholesterol, removes cholesterol from atherosclerotic plaques, then transfers the cholesterol to LDL and VLDL using cholesterol ester transport protein (CETP). From here, the cholesterol is taken back into the liver, as LDLs are reabsorbed.

As I have written many times, in many different places, if you believe this is what happens, you truly will believe anything. In my earlier book *The Great Cholesterol Con* I opined, without any hint of sarcasm, that attempts to raise HDL would have exactly, and precisely, no effect on heart disease because the underlying concept was the finest, highest-quality 100 per cent baloney. But many people ignored me completely. Can you believe it? They felt that raising HDL with drugs of various kinds would be the next great money-making venture. Sorry, the next great breakthrough in curing CVD.

Four of the largest pharmaceutical companies in the world, employing highly paid scientists, who no doubt claimed to have properly functioning brains, in possession of PhDs and suchlike, spent many billions of dollars running massive clinical trials on several different HDL-raising agents, which were primarily designed to block the action of CETP. Well, they could have saved themselves a whole heap of money if they had listened to me. I know that the most irritating and off-putting four words in the English language are, in this order, 'I told you so.' But sometimes the need to say them is irresistible.

Almost ten years after I mocked the concept of HDL-raising agents, we have the following comment about the success of the latest CETP inhibitor, called evacetrapib: 'Steve Nissen, chairman of cardiovascular medicine at Cleveland Clinic, said: "Here we have a paradox. The drug (evacetrapib) more than doubled HDL and lowered LDL levels by as much as many statins – but had no effect on cardiac events."'[1]

In short, a complete and utter failure. In fact, there have been four CETP inhibitors that have gone through clinical trials. They have been such an abject failure that none of them will ever reach the market. The first of the CETP inhibitors to fail, torcetrapib, increased the risk of death from CVD by over 50 per cent. So much for 'good' cholesterol and its wondrous, plaque-chomping skills.

In another delicious twist to this story, researchers have now discovered that HDL can be harmful to some people: 'So-called "good" cholesterol may actually increase heart attack risks in some people, researchers said on Thursday, a discovery that casts fresh doubt on drugs designed to raise it. High-density lipoprotein (HDL) cholesterol is generally associated with reduced heart risks, since it usually offsets the artery-clogging effects of the low-density (LDL) form. But some people have a rare genetic mutation that causes the body to have high levels of HDL and this group, paradoxically, has a higher heart risk, scientists reported in the journal *Science*.'[2]

All of which means, of course, that you can now have 'bad'/'good' or would that be 'good'/'bad' cholesterol. How wonderful. I do love a scientific hypothesis that can flatly contradict itself in two words, yet still manages to be supported by people who honestly think of themselves as scientists. Hint. Money might have something to do with this.

So, what does HDL do, apart from increase the risk of CVD in some people? Well, despite what I have just written HDL does indeed mop up cholesterol. When cells die, the cholesterol released from the cell membrane will float about in the space between the surrounding cells (the interstitial space). HDL is attracted to this and esterifies it (i.e. one cholesterol molecule is stuck to an FFA to form an ester). Once esterified, the HDL can then absorb cholesterol and transfer it back into LDL and VLDL using CETP. In this way, free cholesterol ends up back in the liver as the LDLs are reabsorbed.

What HDL does not do, however, is chisel cholesterol out of atherosclerotic plaques because that would require mechanisms that do not exist in nature (unless HDL is a sentient micro-organism sent by an advanced civilisation from another dimension to cure us of CVD, in which case I shall eat my words).

Having mentioned the most commonly discussed lipoproteins, I need to clear the decks for another lipoprotein, which is hardly ever mentioned. This is somewhat ironic as it is the most interesting lipoprotein of all, and may be the only one that can be directly implicated in CVD. This is lipoprotein (a), usually written as Lp(a).

The story of Lp(a) begins about 40 million years ago, when our ancestors were swinging merrily through the trees eating bananas. This was also when many of the great apes lost the ability to synthesise vitamin C, although this may have happened before great apes even existed, or even bananas, but you get the general idea. Now, there must have been a good reason why our ancestors lost the ability to synthesise vitamin

C, but I am damned if I can find out what it is. The best guess is that some of our forebears got much better at recycling vitamin C, so they needed much less in their diet, and the resources required to synthesise it were better used elsewhere. So, they stopped making it. Perhaps there was a mutation due to a solar flare.

Anyway, because humans cannot synthesise vitamin C, our stores can easily become depleted and we can end up scorbutic, i.e. the condition of lacking vitamin C. Being scorbutic means having scurvy. The major problem in scurvy is that the collagen in our body starts to break down, because vitamin C is required for collagen production.

Collagen, in turn, is a vital support substance throughout the body. It holds most of the tissues in our body together. The bricks in your house, the steel in reinforced concrete, that type of analogy. If collagen fails, everything starts to disintegrate. One of the most serious manifestations of scurvy is within the walls of the blood vessels. If the collagen fails here, the blood vessels start to crack, break open and bleed.

The spectrum of symptoms from scurvy are ghastly. It leads to the formation of brown spots on the skin, spongy gums and bleeding from the nose, mouth and anus. There is also lethargy, immobility and severe depression. In advanced scurvy there are open, festering wounds, loss of teeth and, eventually, death, usually from blood loss.

Now what, you may be asking, has any of this do this have to do with Lp(a)? Well, bleeding to death because you cannot, unlike almost all other animals, synthesise vitamin C represents a pretty serious design flaw. And as with all other badly designed operating systems, evolution came up with a patch. The patch, in this case, was Lp(a).

When cracks develop in blood vessels, Lp(a) is attracted to them, along with all the other things that make up a blood clot. Lp(a) then links to proteins in the artery wall and binds to them very tightly, forming a strong plug that holds back the bleeding. In addition to this, Lp(a) also has another amazing trick up its sleeve. Something so clever that it makes you stand back in awe at the limitless capacity of nature. Almost the moment blood clots form, they are being broken down. But if you completely dissolved the part of the clot that is stuck to a crack on the artery wall, blood would just start leaking out again.

How do you stop this happening? Well, this is where the story takes us back to plasminogen. Just to remind you, plasminogen is the inactive enzyme incorporated into all blood clots as they form. Plasminogen can be converted to plasmin, the active form of the enzyme, that slices clot apart. The enzyme that transforms plasminogen to plasmin is tissue plasminogen activator (tPA).

Lp(a) has a protein attached to it called apolipoprotein A. This protein is virtually identical in structure to plasminogen, apart from one single different amino acid. However, this minute difference is enough to ensure that neither apolipoprotein A, nor the surrounding plasminogen, can be converted to plasmin. So fibrinolysis is blocked and tPA becomes ineffective in those areas of the blood clot where there is a high concentration of Lp(a). All of which means that, when your blood vessels start to break apart in scurvy, Lp(a) not only plugs the gap, it also stops the blood clot that has been formed from being broken down. Because of this, you are more likely to survive in times of vitamin C famine. Thus, you are more likely to have children and pass on your genes. I shall call this concept, in all modesty, 'The theory of evolution by natural selection'.

The other thing you need to know about Lp(a) is that is identical to LDL. Indeed, it *is* LDL, apart from the addition of one extra protein, apolipoprotein A. How remarkable is that?

DIAGRAM 21b

But why did evolution choose to attach apolipoprotein A to LDL, to turn it into Lp(a)? I presume that apolipoprotein A had to be added to something that circulates in the bloodstream, so damage to any blood vessel could easily be reached. Also,

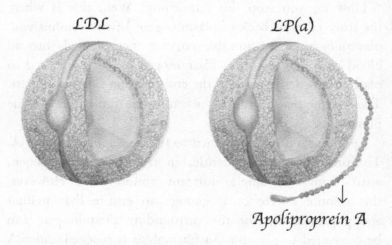

LDL   *LP(a)*

↓

Apoliproprein A

lipoproteins are already designed, in part, as vehicles for apolipoproteins.

Perhaps, most importantly, cholesterol is vital in tissue growth and repair. If you damage any part of the body, you need cholesterol to arrive at the scene and assist in the repair process. Therefore, it makes perfect sense for apolipoprotein A to be attached to a molecule that carries around the most important repair substance in the body – cholesterol. Protection and repair in one package.

What, you may ask, has all this got to do with CVD? Well, although it is true that very few people suffer from scurvy currently, it could still be possible that a chronic, sub-optimal level of vitamin C may lead to low-level cracking of blood vessels. Which means that Lp(a) would be attracted to these areas and then we could have the start of atherosclerotic plaques.

Linus Pauling, a winner of two Nobel Prizes, was the man who very vocally promoted the vitamin C–Lp(a) connection. He believed that CVD was primarily caused by a lack of vitamin C, and to prevent CVD you just need to take a high dose of vitamin C daily. Far more than the daily recommended dose. A cure for CVD ... hoorah.

Of course, this takes the entire idea of what CVD is, and what causes it, off in a completely different direction. A direction whereby blood clots are not only the final event in heart attacks and strokes they are, in fact, the focus of plaque development in the first place, something that was first noted long, long ago: 'Karl von Rokitanksy and Virchow were early investigators who reported that in some instances, the development of atherosclerosis involved early vessel wall injury, thrombosis, and the incorporation of thrombi into the vessel wall. In 1887, Welch gave a clear description of arterial thrombi based on the experiments of a number of investigators, showing that they began as platelet-rich thrombi and are then transformed into masses rich in fibrin. Much later, these observations were reinforced by Duguid, Morgan, More, Haust and French.'[3]

Now that would be a thing, would it not? Plaques are simply blood clots that build up one on top of another, changing in structure and appearance over time ... surely not? In two words, surely so. But how could you ever prove that Linus Pauling was right? Get a few hundred people, completely deplete them of vitamin C and then wait to see if atherosclerosis develops. Well, I suppose there is a distinct danger that they would all die of scurvy first, which would prove very little one way or another.

An additional problem is that I can't see an ethics committee giving such a study the thumbs up. Let us deliberately make hundreds of people scorbutic and see what happens – what could possibly go wrong?

In reality you cannot do experiments like this on human beings, which means that if you are going to study the effect of vitamin C depletion on atherosclerosis, you first need to find an animal to study. Clearly, you need to find an animal unable to synthesise vitamin C, one where you can run down vitamin C stores relativity quickly. That rules out most of the great apes, where depletion would take months, and where you also have other major ethical issues in doing such experiments. I can see the angrily waved placards now.

Step forward the humble guinea pig. Yes, guinea pigs cannot synthesise vitamin C either, and that makes them the ideal experimental animal. So, what happens if you make a guinea pig scorbutic? As far as I am aware this experiment has only been done once, almost sixty years ago, by a man called G.C. Willis.

Willis got a group of guinea pigs and put them on a vitamin C-free diet to deplete their vitamin C stores, and then immediately injected 12 of them with vitamin C to reverse the depletion. None of the 12 developed any measurable atherosclerosis. However, the remaining scorbutic guinea pigs rapidly developed atherosclerosis. When I say rapidly, I mean within days. I think this point is worth repeating. If you make a guinea pig scorbutic, it will develop plaques, identical to those found in human arteries, within days.

Willis then started feeding his scorbutic guinea pigs vitamin C again. He found that the lipid-filled plaques rapidly disappeared and explained that: 'The results of this investigation indicate that early lesions of atherosclerosis are quickly reabsorbed. The stages of this process are first a fading of lipid staining in the region of the internal elastic membrane with later a disappearance of all extracellular fat. Active phagocytosis (ingestion) of lipid by macrophage occurs, and when these macrophages finally disappear no evidence of the lesion remains.'[4]

To put it more simply, Willis found that if you remove vitamin C from the guinea pigs' diet, they develop lipid-filled atherosclerotic plaques within days. If you then add vitamin C to the diet, the plaques rapidly disappear, again within days. The process of removal appears to be that the lipid is ingested (phagocytosed) by a type of white blood cell, the macrophage.

Ironically, the current thinking is that lipid-filled macrophages are an important cause of atherosclerosis because such macrophages are often found in plaques. This is what you call getting cause and effect exactly and precisely the wrong way around. Macrophages are not causing plaques, they are trying to get rid of them. Why else would they be there? To rush in and commit suicide?

Willis also found that if you let the plaques grow for too long, it is far more difficult to get rid of them. They appear to become established, as chronic plaques. He said, 'More advanced lesions are considerably more resistant to reversal.

Extensive lipid deposits clear in some parts of plaque but islands of intensely staining lipid persists in other parts. The macrophage response to such areas is only slight.'

So, it seems that, in guinea pigs at least, if you don't get rid of the plaque/thrombus pretty much straight away, you don't get rid of them at all. Or maybe Willis didn't wait long enough to see what happened over months or even years, although my childhood memory of guinea pigs is that they tend to drop dead at the slightest excuse, so a long-term study may be tricky. 'Blast, another one gone.'

Of course, this was an experiment on guinea pigs not humans, so we must be careful not to extrapolate too far, but note that extrapolating from cholesterol overfeeding studies on rabbits, to humans, was one of the main triggers that started the entire diet/heart hypothesis in the first place. Pity they didn't start with guinea pigs and vitamin C. If they had done so, I suspect research into CVD would now be in a completely different place.

Having said this, Willis had studied humans. Not many, only sixteen. Ten people with identified atherosclerotic plaques were given vitamin C and six were not. Sorry, I do not know the dose. Of the ten treated with vitamin C, the plaques got bigger in three, stayed the same in one and reduced in size in six. Of the six not given vitamin C, three remained the same and in three the plaques got bigger. Interesting, but hardly cast-iron proof of anything.

So, what do we know? First, that animals which cannot synthesise vitamin C are at risk of developing scurvy, causing blood vessels to crack open and bleed. Second, that Lp(a) is present in the bloodstream of animals – including humans who cannot synthesise vitamin C – and its role is to plug the cracks that form in arteries. And third, Lp(a) is associated with a much higher rate of CVD; '... elevated Lp(a) levels associate robustly and specifically with increased CVD risk. The association is continuous in shape without a threshold and does not depend on high levels of LDL or non-HDL cholesterol, or on the levels or presence of other cardiovascular risk factors.'[5]

At this point, you may be wondering why you have never heard of Lp(a) before? I suspect because the pharmaceutical industry has not found any way to bring the level down. In truth you can lower it, if not by a great deal, with niacin (vitamin B3) but there are no patents available on vitamins so there is no real money to be made here. Instead of marketing hype we have deafening silence all round.

And where does this information about vitamin C and Lp(a) take us? To my mind it opens new lines of investigation that could turn the conventional thinking about CVD on its head. Unfortunately, if you are a mainstream medical 'expert' it means nothing at all and gets ignored, which is precisely what has happened. There is almost zero interest in researching vitamin C, or Lp(a), or any combination in CVD.

I believe that this inertia is compounded by the fact that the conventional view of the role of vitamins in disease, of any sort, is deemed as 'woo-woo medicine', on a par with homeopathy and crystal therapy. Apparently, 'proper' researchers should have nothing to do with vitamins or their effects on anything, but this is clearly bonkers. Recently, vitamin C has been found to be enormously beneficial in treating sepsis, which used to be called blood poisoning. Sepsis has a frighteningly high mortality rate. It is one of the most serious medical conditions there is, and anything that can improve survival in sepsis cannot be written off as 'woo-woo medicine'. Just read this report from PulmCCM.

After hundreds of trials failing to show benefit of drug treatments for sepsis, could a simple, cheap and effective treatment – high-dose vitamin C – be hiding in plain sight? A respected leader in critical care medicine thinks so, and his hospital system is all in.

Vitamin C (ascorbic acid) is depleted during sepsis. That might be bad, because ascorbic acid helps maintain the integrity of the endothelium, and is required for the production of catecholamines and cortisol: hormones needed for survival from shock ...

The renowned Dr Paul Marik et al will soon publish in *Chest* their own small before-and-after unblinded study, born of an anecdote that should intrigue any intensivist: three patients with 'fulminant sepsis ... almost certainly destined to die' from shock and organ failure, infused with vitamin C and moderate dose hydrocortisone out of desperation. All three patients recovered quickly and left the ICU in days, 'with no residual organ dysfunction'. [ICU = intensive care unit]

Inspired by that experience, they went on to enroll and treat 47 septic patients with a cocktail of *1.5 g vitamin C IV (intravenous) every 6 hours, hydrocortisone 50 mg IV every 6 hours, and thiamine 200 mg IV every 12 hours* (thiamine has potential benefits in septic shock). Controls were 47 patients matched in baseline characteristics.

Hospital mortality was 4 of 47 (8.5%) in those treated with the cocktail, compared to 19 of 47 (40%) in those not

... Renal function reportedly improved in all patients with acute kidney injury.[6]

My goodness, it turns out that vitamin C is more effective in sepsis than any antibiotic yet discovered. It saves lives in the most serious medical condition known – fulminant sepsis, a.k.a. septic shock. (I wonder if it would work with Ebola ... it should definitely help.)

What has been the impact on the wider medical profession of this finding? Have a wild guess and watch the tumbleweed blowing, wolves howling in a lonely snow-covered scene. Nothing stirs, not even a mouse. Who disturbs my slumbers? But if your loved one is lying in intensive care, severely ill from septic shock, you may want to ask the doctor if they would care to try administering a cocktail of vitamin C, vitamin B1 and hydrocortisone, which could improve chances of recovery from 60 to 93.5 per cent. I can imagine the response. You will be hurled out of the hospital for daring to suggest such a stupid thing. 'Vitamins!' (Think Edith Evans as Lady Bracknell, but she ain't exclaiming 'handbag'.)

How does vitamin C help in sepsis? To answer this you first need to ask, what it is that kills you with sepsis? The really deadly substances in sepsis are the exotoxins produced by bacteria that are multiplying in the bloodstream. They attack the endothelial cells that line your blood vessels. Once attacked, the endothelial cells start to malfunction, losing their anticoagulant (blood-clot prevention) function. This causes blood clots to form throughout the body, which clog the blood vessels in organs, such as the kidneys, liver and lungs, leading to multi-organ failure, shortly followed by death. The technical term for widespread blood clotting is disseminated intravascular coagulation (DIC). Yes, back with blood clotting and the endothelium again.

It seems that exotoxins strip vitamin C out of endothelial cells, which severely weakens them. Or, perhaps the endothelial cells burn through vitamin C stores as they desperately attempt to protect themselves. Thus, if you add high doses of vitamin C to standard treatment, the endothelial cells can keep up the fight for longer, allowing the antibiotics to kill off the bacteria before their exotoxins kill you. This is rather like what happens with Lp(a) and scurvy, although that happens on a much longer timescale. If you become vitamin C deficient, Lp(a) will not keep you alive forever but it will protect the lining of your arteries until you can find more vitamin C.

At this point, it may seem that I come a very long way from describing lipoproteins to this discussion about the use of vitamin C in sepsis. But I wanted to reinforce the point that everything in the body is extremely complex and inter-related.

We have been spoon-fed the story that LDL is simply a little sphere that floats about in the bloodstream and transports cholesterol into cells. However, when you really start to study lipoproteins, you find that they are far more complex, with many more functions in the human body than you may have thought possible. LDL, for example, is basically Lp(a), or vice versa, which has multiple roles in blood clotting and arterial protection.

It certainly does not end here. There are a couple of other facts about LDL that are highly relevant. LDL binds to exotoxins as they are released from bacteria, which also protects the endothelium from damage. Because of this, people with higher LDL levels are much less likely to end up in hospital with infections.[7]

In animal models, mice that have been genetically manipulated to have very high LDL levels are highly resistant to bacterial toxins/exotoxins. In the type of experiment that you cannot do on humans, for obvious reasons, you can calculate the dose of an agent that will kill 50 per cent of the animals taking it. This is called the lethal dose fifty, or LD_{50}.

If you inject an exotoxin into mice with very high LDL levels, the LD_{50} is eight times higher than that required in 'normal' mice. That is, you need eight times the dose of exotoxin to kill 50 per cent of the mice, which is an enormously powerful and important effect.[8]

However, the benefits of LDL do not stop there. LDL does not merely neutralise exotoxins, it also binds to the bacteria themselves, and holds them in place to be attacked and killed by white blood cells. So, you could say that LDL is a form of antibiotic agent.[9] This is probably why children with Smith-Lemli-Opitz syndrome, who have very low LDL levels, are far more likely to suffer from recurrent and life-threatening infections.

This could also explain why a genetic study done in the Netherlands found that people with familial hypercholesterolaemia (FH) lived longer than anyone else in the nineteenth century. A protection that disappeared, indeed reversed, in the first half of the twentieth century, before changing again. Today, those with FH have the same life expectancy as everyone else.

'We found that the excess mortality from familial hypercholesterolaemia varied over time. In the 19th century, mortality seemed lower than in the general population. It rose after 1915, reached a maximum during the 1950s, and decreased thereafter ... such large variation in mortality in two directions (over time and within generations) indicates that the disorder has strong interactions with environmental factors.'[10]

During the nineteenth century, infections were *the* leading cause of death, so if you had a high level of LDL, this would confer significant advantages. Then, as clean water and improved sanitation arrived, followed by antibiotics, protection against infections would have been less important for survival, and having FH would be less beneficial.

Indeed, if FH affords protection against infection, this may explain why FH continues to exist as a genetic condition rather than dying out. It also probably explains why a high cholesterol level becomes increasingly beneficial as we get older. After the age of around sixty, the higher your LDL level is, the longer you will live because infections become an increasingly common cause of death.[11]

The final thing I need to add about lipoproteins is that HDL has quite potent anticoagulant effects.'... our studies confirm that *fresh HDL possesses anticoagulant cofactor activity*, as we previously reported. Understanding the components of HDL and the mechanisms by which this beneficial property occur could lead to novel therapeutic approaches to the prevention of venous thrombosis.'[12] Yes, HDL is an anticoagulant, and this raises a further possibility that 'good' cholesterol does not provide protection due to any effect on cholesterol. It is because it stops blood clotting.

I will end this chapter with a final issue for you to ponder. If you find LDL in atherosclerotic plaques, are you finding LDL or Lp(a)? And how could you possibly tell the difference? They both contain exactly the same amount of cholesterol and triglyceride and they both have apo lipoprotein B-100 attached. Tricky to tell which is which, especially if you don't bother specifically looking for apolipoprotein A.

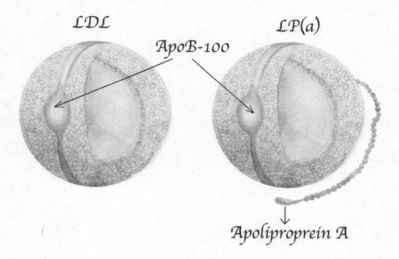

In fact, specifically looking for apolipoprotein A in atherosclerotic plaques has been studied, as far as I can establish, precisely once in the history of medical research, and guess what. When it was looked for it was found – at high levels.[13] How else do you think those guinea pigs ended up with atherosclerotic plaques in their arteries, within days of being made scorbutic? What do you think was present in those plaques? Fat, cholesterol, LDL or Lp(a)?

CHAPTER 9

Cholesterol Lowering Without Statins

⬤▭

Although statins now bestride the world of cholesterol like a colossus, over the years there have been many other attempts to lower LDL, and/or raise HDL, using a wide range of different drugs. I think it is important to look at them in some detail, as this can help to shed light in dark places. Namely, does lowering cholesterol work.

In order of when they first appeared we have:

- 1955 vitamin B3 (nicotinic acid)
- 1958 clofibrate, followed by other fibrates, e.g. gemfibrozil, fenofibrate
- 1959 triparanol (MER/29), followed by probucol in 1982
- 1973 cholestryamine (possibly developed in 1900, but clearly not launched then); also closely related, colestipol

- 1987 lovastatin, followed by many other statins
- 2002 ezetimibe (descendant of cholestyramine)
- 2005, various drugs to raise HDL (the 'rapibs')
- 2015 PSCK9 inhibitor, proprotein convertase subtilisin/kexin type 9 inhibitor

There may have been others that never saw the light of day because, until 2005, if you carried out a clinical trial and it was negative there was no requirement to publish it. You could just bury it and move on. So, who knows how many LDL-lowering agents have been tested over the years and failed to have any effect? None, ten, 100… your guess is as good as mine.

In addition to LDL-lowering agents, as briefly described earlier, there was a drive to find drugs that raised HDL and thus lower the risk of CVD. There have been four major ones, the rapibs:

- torcetrapib
- dalcetrapib
- evacetrapib
- anacetrapib

These are the drugs that time forgot, or will forget, despite thousands of patients being enrolled in clinical trials, and hundreds and hundreds of millions of research dollars spent.

Torcetrapib was the first of the rapibs to report results. It raised HDL by about 60 per cent, and increased the overall mortality rate by about 50 per cent. Dalcetrapib did nothing, either positive or negative. The latest of them, anacetrapib, managed to scrape some positive findings but Merck decided not to bother marketing it at all, as the benefits were so weak, some might say non-existent. To quote a Merck spokesman: 'After comprehensive evaluation, we have concluded that the clinical profile for anacetrapib does not support regulatory filings'. Which is code for 'Oh, bollocks to it.'[1]

The main reason for mentioning the rapibs is not just to confirm that raising HDL does nothing. It is to highlight the fact that, inadvertently, one of the trials managed to leave the LDL hypothesis standing naked in the rain. Evacetrapib raised HDL by 120 per cent and also lowered LDL by 37 per cent, which is more than most statins manage. Yet the impact on CVD was exactly and precisely zero. To quote Steven Nissen, who ran the trial: 'the results can't be explained because the study was too small or because too few heart attacks and strokes occurred. The drug didn't work.'[2] But in a later discussion he went on to make an extraordinary statement at the end of this passage, taken from *Cardiology News*:

'We were astonished by the LDL effects in our study. Conventional wisdom says that a 37% drop in LDL cholesterol should translate into a benefit in high-risk patients,' he noted. 'This reinforces the concept that mechanism matters. Surrogate endpoints are not a replacement for clinical endpoints. We need to understand more about LDL cholesterol. We thought that [lowering LDL cholesterol] was straightforward, but it's not.

'The most important lesson from this study is the hazard of making [efficacy] assumptions based on surrogate endpoints,' said Dr Frederick Masoudi, a professor of medicine at the University of Colorado in Aurora. 'The way you get to a lower LDL cholesterol level is important.

'There are two hypotheses to explain the results: Either lowering LDL cholesterol was beneficial but something else evacetrapib did caused toxicity' and counterbalanced the benefit of LDL cholesterol lowering, 'or it matters how you lower LDL cholesterol,' said Dr Nissen, chairman of the department of cardiovascular medicine at the Cleveland Clinic. *I personally think it's the latter, that mechanism [of LDL cholesterol lowering] counts,'* he said in an interview.'[3] [My emphasis]

By the way, a surrogate end-point is a measurement, e.g. blood pressure, blood cholesterol or blood sugar levels. It is assumed that lowering these surrogate end-points is beneficial, and will result in clinical benefits, e.g. reduction in CVD. However, this is often not the case. Obviously pharmaceutical companies far prefer to 'treat' surrogate end-points, then claim this will provide clinical benefits. Because while you can lower the blood pressure in an hour, it takes many years, and hundreds of millions of dollars, to run a trial looking at proper outcomes.

In this case, the surrogate end-point was lowering LDL by 37 per cent. According to the cholesterol/LDL hypothesis, this should have resulted in major benefits concerning heart attacks and strokes. In fact, it resulted in no benefit all, which contradicts everything everyone believes about LDL and, of course, the entire cholesterol hypothesis.

What was the preferred method of ignoring this result? Normally, the opinion leaders call findings like this a paradox, and then it is allowed to gather dust until everyone forgets it ever happened. This time, though, we have been given an explanation. The mechanism of LDL lowering is what counts.

Sit back, close your eyes and swirl that thought around in your mind. Examine it from all angles. Take your time. Construct the statement another way. The level of LDL that you achieve with treatment does not matter, what matters is *how* you managed to get it down to that level.

Try again. Of course, I cannot tell you how to think. You will, no doubt, find other ways to deconstruct and reconstruct that comment. Perhaps you prefer to pay attention to Dr Masoudi who phrased it thus: 'The way you get to a lower LDL cholesterol is important.' It is at times like this that I normally reach for a copy of *Alice's Adventures in Wonderland* to find that Lewis Carroll had already said it first, and far better, than me.

> Alice laughed: 'There's no use trying,' she said; 'one can't believe impossible things.'
>
> 'I daresay you haven't had much practice,' said the Queen. 'When I was younger, I always did it for half an hour a day. Why, sometimes I've believed as many as six impossible things before breakfast.

Gentle mockery aside, I do not understand those statements by Masoudi and Nissen, which seem devoid of any logic. I wonder what happened in the lecture theatre where they came up with this explanation. I imagine everyone just nodded sagely and wrote down, 'The way you lower LDL is the important thing, not the level you achieve,' using an expensive pen specially purchased to inscribe such comments. They probably underlined the statement carefully, whilst nodding wisely to themselves. Then thought no more of it. Nothing to see here, move along.

Patient: 'So my cholesterol level is now normal.'

Doctor: 'Yes, but I am afraid it was not brought down in an approved manner, so it is of no benefit to you whatsoever.'

Had I been there, I may have raised my hand to ask, 'But does this not flatly contradict the cholesterol hypothesis?' Which is exactly what I did, many years ago, when the results of the Medical Research Council's (MRC) trial on mild to moderate blood pressure lowering were presented at a cardiology conference in Scotland.

This was a landmark trial, the first ever large-scale placebo-controlled clinical study to ask the question. Does lowering mildly raised blood pressure work? Mildly raised, in those days, was anything over 160/110 which, today, would result in you being rushed into hospital with malignant hypertension. I exaggerate, but only slightly.

In the MRC trial, 17,354 patients were recruited and there were 85,572 patient years of observation. After all this, there were 248 deaths in the treated group and 253 deaths in the placebo group. It turned out that treating nearly 9,000 people for five years resulted in five fewer deaths. That equates to very nearly 9,000 years of treatment to delay one death. There was absolutely no difference in CV mortality.[4]

My first thought was, 'Crikey, what a complete and utter waste of time.' I raised my hand and gently suggested (I was young and naïve at the time) that this trial seemed to suggest that lowering blood pressure was not really very effective. Or perhaps I wasn't so timid. The temperature in the lecture theatre suddenly plummeted about 30 degrees.

Now, whilst statins may be the most prescribed group of

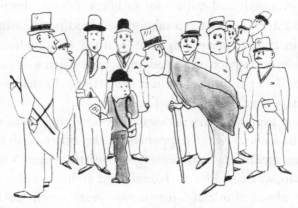

medicines in history, there are still more people taking various blood pressure lowering agents in total. So, you can see what impact the MRC trial had. Which reminds me of Winston Churchill's 'Men occasionally stumble over the truth, but most of them pick themselves up and hurry off as if nothing had happened.'

Oh, but things have changed, haven't they? Well, a far more recent review looked at treating blood pressure from 140–159mmHg. This is a significantly lower level than studied in the MRC trial, but it represents the point at which your doctor will now recommend that you need to take blood pressure lowering tablets, for the rest of your life. This review came to the following conclusion: 'At a period of four to five years follow up, *no differences were seen in mortality, cardiovascular events, Coronary artery disease, or stroke.* Approximately 9% more patients in the treatment arms withdrew due to medication side effects.'[5] They also put it another way: 'None were helped (preventing death, stroke, heart disease, or cardiovascular events).' However, they added that '1 in 12 were harmed (medication side effects and stopped the drug).'

So, no benefit and quite a lot of harm. Almost the perfect medical intervention. Keep taking the blood pressure tablets, chaps. In truth, I have long since learned that evidence has absolutely no impact on the adamantine carapace of medical practice. Belief trumps evidence, every time. Evidence-based medicine – 'you're 'aving a larf, mate'.

Having somewhat drifted away from lowering LDL, I shall return to look at what happened to the other cholesterol-lowering agents that have emerged over the years. Vitamin B3/niacin was the first to launch and it has continued to wander about aimlessly for many years, without being withdrawn, partly because vitamin B3 not only lowers LDL, it also boosts HDL and lowers VLDL. Also, as it is a vitamin, you cannot really withdraw it from human consumption or we would all die.

More recently, niacin been used in combination with statins to see if it can provide an additional benefit. There were the HPS2-THRIVE and AIM-HIGH trials, both very big and long lasting. Both reported as recently as 2011 and 2013, and both failed to show any benefit at all. The underlying dream was that if you added niacin to a statin, you could market this as a 'combination drug' and extend various patents for many years. Sorry chaps, not to be.

After the failure of vitamin B3 came the fibrates. Clofibrate first, followed by gemfibrozil and fenofibrate. Clofibrate was discontinued in 2002 because it increased the risk of cancer, as did the other fibrates. In addition, none of them had managed to demonstrate any benefit on overall or heart disease mortality.

Triparanol (MER/29) then emerged, followed by probucol. These drugs, like statins, blocked cholesterol synthesis, although towards the very end of the cholesterol synthesis pathway. However, they were both rapidly withdrawn after causing very serious adverse effects, such as cataracts, skin damage and neuropathy, conditions that are also, it should be noted, associated with statins.

Then we moved on to colestipol and cholestyramine, which both work in pretty much the same way. They bind to bile/cholesterol in the guts and stop it being reabsorbed. More cholesterol then must be directed from the liver to become bile and this, in turn, lowers the cholesterol/LDL level. More recently ezetimibe was launched, which does pretty much the same thing, but with fewer side effects.

Did these earlier drugs work at all? Well, as with most things in medical research, that rather depends on what you decide to measure. The WHO trial on colestipol lasted over five years and had slightly more than 15,000 subjects, looking at the overall mortality. Of those taking colestipol, there were 128 deaths. Of those taking placebo, 87 deaths. There was no difference in fatal CVD.

Despite this failure, a major follow-up trial using cholestyramine was done. Called the Coronary Primary Prevention Trial (CPPT), it lasted more than seven years and was published in 1984. While 500,000 people were initially screened, this figure was whittled this down to 3,800 men, half taking the drug, half the placebo. The average cholesterol level (total cholesterol) was 7.55mmol/l (292mg/dl). (In the US they use a different system of measurement for cholesterol. It is milligrams per decilitre mg/dl, not mmol/l.) This level, as you may have noticed, is very high.[6]

The CPPT trial was reported in many ways. However, I shall keep things as simple as possible by focusing on overall and CV mortality. That is, how many people died, of anything, and how many people died specifically of CVD, which is supposed to be improved by lowering LDL. (Those running clinical trials, and their pharmaceutical company sponsors, truly hate using absolute and CVD as an end-point, unless they unexpectedly improve, in which case you never hear the end of it.)

Looking at the overall mortality, the result of the CPPT was that there was no difference, at all, in overall mortality between the two groups. So of 1,900 men, with extremely high cholesterol levels, treated for 7.4 years, not one lived a day longer. If we look at CV mortality, the figures are pretty much the same, although eight more people died of CVD in the placebo than in the treatment group. To put it another way, for every 1,763 years of treatment, just one CV death was delayed; note, I did *not* say 'prevented', which I will explain later.

Of course, this was hailed as a major triumph around the world. The cholesterol hypothesis was proven, at last. 'The major medical journals around the world hailed the results of the trial as finally providing the rationale for treating hypercholesterolemia. *The Medical Journal of Australia* featured a lead article by Leon A. Simons titled "The lipid hypothesis is proven".'[7]

Time magazine's report ran: 'Cholesterol is proved deadly ... Lowering cholesterol levels markedly reduces the incidence of fatal heart attacks.' They just forgot to add, 'you need to live for 1,763 years to see a benefit'.

Was this trial a success? Did it prove the cholesterol hypothesis? In my opinion, if you think that trial proved anything, you need to go and lie down in a darkened room for a while – about 1,763 years should do it. I suppose we all see what we want to see. Group-think confirmation bias adds to desperate hope. Imagine if you had to treat people with penicillin for 1,763 years before anyone benefited, and you still failed to save a single life. Whoop-de-doo.

Of course, with the arrival of statins, all arguments were simply brushed aside. Statins were not only much more effective at lowering LDL than anything that had gone before, they also managed to do something nothing else had achieved up to that point. They lowered both CVD and overall mortality. Eminent cholesterol sceptics, such as Professor Michael Oliver, ended up writing an editorial in the *British Medical Journal* (*The BMJ*) entitled 'Lower patients' cholesterol now.' He too had been seduced by the dark side.

Along with Oliver, almost everyone who had previously been sceptical of the cholesterol hypothesis conceded defeat at this point. Here we had a new class of drugs that did exactly what they said on the tin. They were specifically designed to lower LDL, which they did. They also reduced the risk of CVD. End of. Only a complete fool could argue against evidence as clear cut as this ... Who, me?

Before statins came along I had dismissed the cholesterol hypothesis as scientific nonsense. However, I must admit the arrival of statins did cause me to pause and rethink. I think it is safe to say that, prior to the arrival of statins, the cholesterol hypothesis had not been proven one way or the other by the drug trials, and not for the sake of trying. But statins shifted the tectonic plates and the opposition was driven from the battleground. Then I found a group of scientists and researchers on the internet known as The International Network of Cholesterol Sceptics (THINCS), set up by Dr Uffe Ravnskov, a Swedish doctor and researcher. Hoorah, I was not alone. Almost everyone in THINCS has a different idea on what causes CVD, but we are all united around one idea: that a raised LDL/cholesterol does not cause CVD.

Of course, statins do not represent the end of this story. After statins, there have been two new cholesterol-lowering drugs, or drug classes, that have launched: ezetimibe and PCSK9 inhibitors. How have they fared?

Ezetimibe is, essentially, an updated version of cholestyramine. It binds to bile salts/cholesterol in the gut and removes cholesterol from the body. It is simple to take. Whilst cholestyramine was a powder that had to be sprinkled on food, or mixed with water, and it looked and tasted unpleasant, ezetimibe is a simple pill with very few adverse effects. It gained approval from the regulatory authorities without any difficulty. It was launched and marketed with great success, purely on the basis that it lowered LDL levels. There was no data to prove that it had any beneficial effect on anything – other than LDL levels, that good old surrogate end-point.

In fact, the saga of ezetimibe is a tale of a great battle that unfolded, hidden from the public and almost everyone in the medical profession. But for those of us who knew what was going on, it was all quite ferocious, and remains so – camouflaged by the cloak of overt scientific respectability.

At times, I think the scientific world is like a well-tended garden. All seems calm and tranquil, but there is a fight-to-the-death battle for supremacy. Plant A is trying to slowly strangle plant B. Plant C is sucking the water out of the ground to cause plant D to die of thirst. Plant E is growing thick leaves to block the sunlight needed by plant F. But when you sit on your deckchair, all appears peaceful.

Anyway, what was this great, silent war, of which the world

was, and remains, blissfully unaware? It was the surrogate end-point war. More specifically, does lowering LDL with any medication, other than statins, reduce the risk of CVD? Some of the main weapons used were very familiar: incomprehensible statistics, careful end-point manipulation and money.

Prior to the launch of statins, lowering cholesterol with all previous drugs had been, pretty much, a busted flush. Some slight improvement on non-fatal CV events but *nothing* on CV mortality. In many cases overall morality had gone in completely the wrong direction, by which I mean it had increased.

To make matters worse – in my case better – ezetimibe then ran into very stormy waters. A clinical trial had, eventually, been done, the results being published in 2008 (note in this quote that the brand name of ezetimibe in the US is Zetia).

A clinical trial of Zetia, a cholesterol-lowering drug prescribed to about 1 million people a week, failed to show that the drug has any medical benefits, Merck and Schering-Plough said on Monday ...

While Zetia lowers cholesterol by 15 per cent to 20 per cent in most patients, no trial has ever shown that it can reduce heart attacks and strokes – or even that it reduces the growth of the fatty plaques in arteries that can cause heart problems.

This trial was designed to show that Zetia could reduce the growth of those plaques. Instead, the plaques actually grew almost twice as fast in patients taking Zetia along with Zocor than in those taking Zocor alone. Dr Steven Nissen, the chairman of cardiology at the Cleveland Clinic, said the results were 'shocking.'

'Patients should not be prescribed Zetia unless all other cholesterol drugs have failed,' he said.

'This is as bad a result for the drug as anybody could have feared,' Dr Nissen said. 'Millions of patients may be taking a drug that has no benefits for them, raising their risk of heart attacks and exposing them to potential side effects,' he said.[8]

Oops. Another thing that needs to be mentioned is that the results of this trial were not initially published, some claiming that they were suppressed by the companies involved. They were only released when the US Congress took an interest in the matter. 'Details of the ENHANCE trial, which examined the hypothesis that a combination of simvastatin and ezetimibe would lower low density lipoprotein (LDL) cholesterol and ameliorate atherosclerosis were finally published in the *New England Journal of Medicine* after a press release in January of 2008 – 20 months after the trial had finished and *pressure from the United States Congress to publish* the results in a peer-reviewed journal.'[9]

Hmmmmm. Yet another spectacular fail for a cholesterol-lowering agent. One medical commentator summed things up well. 'The fact that LDL-C lowering by the agents used, either in combination, or independently, had no effect on atheroma reduction has been interpreted by many observers as continuing evidence that LDL-C lowering does not confer clinical benefits. The ENHANCE trial, in fact, enhances the conclusions from most of the major statin trials that there is no association between the degree of total cholesterol or LDL-C lowering and the CHD survival rate.'[10]

Not long afterwards, the American College of Cardiology

(ACC), the AHA and the National Heart, Lung and Blood Institute (NHLBI), which are the holy trinity, the three most powerful and influential bodies involved in CV medicine, came out with their revised Adult Treatment Panel guidance on lowering blood cholesterol. These guidelines carry the power of a papal edict amongst cardiologists worldwide. The headline change ran: 'New Cholesterol Guidelines Abandon LDL Targets', explaining, 'Gone are the recommended LDL- and non-HDL–cholesterol targets, specifically those that ask physicians to treat patients with cardiovascular disease to less than 100 mg/dL or the optional goal of less than 70 mg/d. According to the expert panel, there is *simply no evidence* from randomised, controlled clinical trials to support treatment to a specific target.'[11]

Gosh, now there's a to-do. The tectonic plates had shifted again. Those of us who had been arguing for many years that there was no evidence from the clinical trials that there was any correlation between the degree of LDL lowering achieved and clinical benefit – and who had been ridiculed for saying so, for many years – appeared fully vindicated. Indeed, whilst ezetimibe lowered LDL it accelerated plaque development. Was the LDL hypothesis now dead? Of course, no one dared come straight out and say this.

Here, for instance is the comment by Donald Lloyd Jones, co-chair of the Guidelines Committee: 'There have been no clinical trials in which they've taken an approach where they've titrated medication dosing to achieve a certain LDL level. We just haven't had those trials designed or performed yet. So we just couldn't endorse that kind of approach. And yet, we're not abandoning the measurement of LDL cholesterol, because it's perhaps our best marker of understanding whether patients are going to achieve as much benefit as they can for the dose of statin they can tolerate ...'

So, according to Dr Jones, there is no point in 'treating to target', and despite this, they are going to recommend measuring the LDL levels when you are on treatment anyway. This statement makes absolutely no damned sense at all to me.

The reality is that – statins aside, and it was increasingly argued that they did not work by lowering LDL – from 2008 until 2014 there truly was no evidence from anywhere that lowering LDL provided any benefit. In fact, the ENHANCE trial made it look as though it may be doing harm. The mainstream had reached what I like to call the 'Wile E. Coyote dilemma'. They had run off the edge of a precipice and into thin air, with only the mad thrashing of limbs to keep them airborne.

Gentle readers, was this to be the end of the cholesterol hypothesis? No, of course not. This is the cliff edge that does not, cannot exist. Everyone must keep running furiously and all will be well. This hypothesis supports too many reputations to be allowed to plummet to its doom.

From the financial point of view, Merck had already made a lot of money out of ezetimibe and it made good business sense to continue to do so for as long as possible. They had combined it with simvastatin as a drug called Vytorin (simvastatin + ezetimibe). This extended the simvastatin patent on the basis that it increased LDL lowering in combination with ezetimibe. This legitimately kept the patent alive. Vytorin was making nearly $2 billion a year in profit in the US alone. My problem is that I do not see any clinical evidence to support the thesis that lowering LDL is beneficial in reducing the risk of heart attacks or strokes.

In addition, lined up and with engines running, were PCSK-9 inhibitors, a new class of drugs for lowering LDL even more dramatically than statins. The world was being readied for their multi-billion-dollar arrival. Sorry, their life-saving arrival.

But a ghost had arrived at this feast. If lowering LDL was simply a surrogate marker, and lowering it meant nothing, these drugs too were going to bomb. They were certainly going to have to show some real clinical benefits, above and beyond LDL lowering. The companies involved believed they could easily convince the authorities that LDL lowering was, essentially, the same as lowering the risk of CVD. No need for any of those outcome studies that cost so much, and take so long, and eat into the life of the patents, a.k.a. 'the happy time, when you can make vast profits'.

Hence the clinical trial called IMPROVE-IT, upon which so much rested. The **IMP**roved **R**eduction of **O**utcomes: **V**ytorin **E**fficacy **I**nternational **T**rial. Horrible, convoluted acronym or not, the IMPROVE-IT trial *was* going to prove beyond any shadow of a doubt that ezetimibe really did work, despite accelerating plaque growth. The detractors were not convinced. Battle was joined again.

IMPROVE-IT did not look at using ezetimibe v placebo. It looked at simvastatin + ezetimibe (Vytorin) v simvastatin alone. It would have been considered unethical not to have a statin arm, as statins are 'proven' to protect against CVD, so you would be withholding a lifesaving medication in one arm of the trial. Now, I am going to look at this trial in rather painstaking detail because it was hailed as a massive success, but there are many things about it that can be criticised, a polite way of saying that in my view it was a complete load of

... Just for starters, this trial was statistically powered to need 10,000 participants. Subsequently the investigators found it necessary to add another 8,000 or so.

POWERING CLINICAL TRIALS

Powering trials means, essentially, having enough participants to achieve statistical significance. Imagine you are doing a trial to find out if a coin will land heads or tails. Your prior assumption is that it will land heads or tails the same number of times. This is the null hypothesis, i.e. there is no difference between heads and tails (unless the coin is biased).

If you toss the coin ten times and get ten heads in a row, have you proved that this coin is biased? Have you disproven the null hypothesis? Well, this sequence could happen by chance, but the odds would be long. In this case, the odds are 1 in 1024.

So, how many times do you need to toss a coin to prove it is or it not biased? Clearly, the more tosses the better, as this will smooth out a run of ten heads or ten tails. However, you need to agree on the point that defines the result as significant; 1 in 20, 100 or 1,000? In clinical trials, 1 in 20 is the accepted figure, and is often written as p (probability) < 0.05, i.e. less than a 5 per cent probability that this could be a chance result.

If you are looking for a relatively small effect in a clinical trial, e.g. a 2 per cent reduction in CV mortality, it is much easier to knock this figure backwards and forwards with a run of chance results than, say, when flipping a coin. You need a lot of 'events' to smooth out random variation 'noise' and see a true signal emerging. So, before the trial starts you must state what difference in events you think you are going to see, and how many events it will take before you can be sure you have disproven the null hypothesis $p < 0.05$. The smaller the difference you expect to see, the bigger the number of participants you need to adequately power the study.

A report by Bruce Patsy and Thomas Lumley of Washington University stated that:

IMPROVE-IT, which has already enrolled 11 000 test subjects – 1000 more than its original target enrolment of 10 000 – will be delayed to accrue 18 000 test participants, the companies say. The trial is designed to detect a reduction in cardiovascular death, non-fatal myocardial infarction, rehospitalisation for unstable angina, coronary revascularisation, or stroke as a primary endpoint.

Merck and Schering-Plough say that the decision to extend enrolment, expected to delay results until 2012 or later, is based on a review of two meta-analyses that led them to reassess their original projection that 2955 cardiac events would be sufficient for analysis. The companies now say that they have 'determined that a total of approximately 5250 [cardiovascular] events would be required to have appropriate power to detect a significant reduction in risk.'

'The decision to extend enrolment of participants in a lipid lowering trial that was set to come to an end in 2011 because the target for enrolments had already been exceeded *is causing controversy.*' [12]

'... is causing controversy'. Well, you don't say. This trial was set to come an end in 2011. It was finally published on 8 June 2015. Several years of delay in completing a clinical trial is never a good sign. It suggests that the word 'swimmingly' was not being used at Merck HQ on a regular basis. One can imagine their staff running about, tearing their hair and beating their breasts mightily.

Now, doubling the number of recruits in a trial, after it has started, may have been done before but I have never heard of it. Then virtually doubling the number of events – remember, an event is a heart attack, stroke or hospital admission with angina, etc. – required from 2,955 to 5,250? What reason was given for doubling the participants 'based on a review of two meta-analyses that led them to reassess their original projection'. These trials cost hundreds of millions to run. Adding 8,000–9,000 more people would cost hundreds of millions more. Delaying a clinical trial is like watching the space shuttle take off, then suddenly realising you haven't enough fuel.

> Mission control: '*Challenger*, this is Houston, we would like you to abort the launch and glide back down, so we can fuel the space shuttle fully.'
> *Challenger* captain: '[insert swear words of choice]'

So, which meta-analyses suddenly emerged that led the investigators to reassess their original projection? They didn't feel the need to share this with anyone else. I have read, and read again, various very boring reports on this matter including 'An update on the Improved Reduction of Outcomes: Vytorin Efficacy International Trial (IMPROVE-IT) design', in the *American Heart Journal*. It contains many thousands of words but to my mind fails to explain anything at all, and most certainly does not mention the two meta-analyses.

That report did, however, include the priceless statement: 'To avoid introducing potential bias in the ongoing trial, we describe the parameters that have yielded the conclusion rather than revealing exact numbers in the calculations. These numbers will, however, be publicly available at the trial's conclusion.'[13]

Really? In what way could revealing the numbers in their calculations make the slightest difference to anyone involved in the trial? How could this possibly introduce bias? There are well-recognised ways to eliminate bias in clinical trials, and keeping the statistical calculations used as a well-guarded secret is not one of them. Hardly anyone would have a chance of understanding them, let alone changing their objective measurements. Can someone please explain to me why this statement is not complete and utter baloney?

Some might also find it extremely surprising that investigators were going to reveal the exact numbers they were using after the trial ended, rather than before it started. It's a bit like someone in a pub quiz announcing they knew the answer to a question, immediately having been told it.

And just to add to the strangeness, those running the IMPROVE-IT trials did not even define how long it was going to last. Were they simply going to wait until they had a total of 5,250 events? Who knows? Of course, if you have to wait too long the statistics can start changing, and not in your favour.

In addition, and very weirdly indeed, one year after it ended, the IMPROVE-IT trial protocol was changed. The trial finished in September 2014, the results were published in the *New England Journal of Medicine* in June 2015[14] and the trial protocol was changed on 29 September 2015. As for the length of the trial ... it 'will continue until a minimum of 5,250 subjects have a primary endpoint event and each subject is followed for a minimum of 2.5 years' was now changed 'up to approximately 9 years'.[15]

Whatever you wish to make of what went on in this trial, it came up with a favourable result. Or did it?

Pop Quiz:
- What was the reduction in overall mortality with ezetimibe?
- What was the reduction in CV mortality with ezetimibe?

Answer, it was the same for both outcomes. Zero. Yes, you read that right. Zero benefit. The actual figures were:

- Death from any cause, simvastatin alone = 1,231
- Death from any cause, simvastatin + ezetimibe = 1,215
- Death from cardiovascular causes, simvastatin alone = 538
- Death from cardiovascular causes, simvastatin + ezetimibe = 537

You may object to me saying there was no benefit at all, but sixteen fewer deaths in 9,000 people over 7.4 years sits comfortably within the boundary of pure chance, and proves nothing at all. Of more interest, as ezetimibe lowers LDL, the single most important outcome where you would hope to see benefit was in CVD. Yet all that happened was an eye-watering *one* fewer death from CVD.

One fewer CV death in 9,000 patients over 7.4 years or one less death after *66,000 years* of treatment.

Despite this, IMPROVE-IT was inevitably described as a 'game changer', as such trials are. As such it was destined to earn vast sums of money. You may wonder how it can possibly be be true that a trial, designed to look at the prevention of CVD was deemed to be positive when there was no difference in overall or CV morality. To most people this might seem to represent the most abject failure.

Oh no, not at all. Because measuring overall mortality and CV mortality was not the sole aim. In fact, this trial was not powered, or expected, to show any difference in these outcomes. The primary end-point, upon which success or failure of this trial rested, was a combined end-point consisting of five separate factors:

- CV death
- MI
- Unstable angina requiring rehospitalisation
- Coronary revascularisation
- Stroke

You may have spotted that CV death *was* one of the end-points. However, clearly it did not need to change for this trial to be considered a success. Indeed, we know it did *not* change, and the trial *was* considered a success. One of the problems about having a quintuple end-point, is that all that is needed is for one of them to show a benefit and the entire combined edifice can be dragged into the hallowed realm of statistical significance.

If I had added 'Patient stubbed toe' to this list, with more people taking only simvastatin rather than vytorin stubbing their toes, I could claim success in my primary end-point of CV death, MI, unstable angina requiring rehospitalisation, coronary revascularisation, stroke and *stubbed toe*. You may say, don't be ridiculous, and I would agree. How can anyone simply add what they like to an end-point and mix it up with clinically important outcomes?

And what of the other outcomes? First, coronary revascularisation, which is essentially inserting a stent to open a narrowed coronary artery. A plumbing job. The first thing to say is that this is not actually a clinical end-point, it is a clinical *decision*, usually made by a cardiologist. You cannot *suffer* a coronary revascularisation decision. (Well, you probably can, but that is a different issue entirely.)

So, we actually have four clinical outcomes:

- CV death
- MI
- Unstable angina requiring rehospitalisation
- Stroke

And one, non-clinical outcome ...

- Coronary revascularisation

Just to repeat, if any of these five outcomes changed sufficiently, it could drag the entire combined end-point towards statistical significance, even if none of the other events changed at all.

First question. Why would a cardiologist decide to put in a stent? Well, one the most important reasons is because someone has just suffered an MI and been admitted to hospital, whereupon they will be rushed into the cath lab to be revascularised. So, if there are an increased number of MIs, there will inevitably be more coronary revascularisations – by default.

This means that you are immediately in danger of double counting events. So, 100 MIs lead to, say, 70 revascularisations. Thus, 100 MIs will create 170 different events to be counted, even if they are just two consequences of the same event; one clinical, one procedural. But it gets more complicated than that. If you have a revascularisation, it can cause a subsequent MI. This can happen in up to 50 per cent of people having revascularisation – worst case scenario – which means that you can now triple count, with one event becoming three. First you have an MI (one end-point), you are then taken to the cath lab for a stent (two end-points) and then you have another MI due to the procedure (three end-points). But all this depends on what, and how, you decide to count and what you decide to censor.

Furthermore, a cardiologist may decide to put in a stent after an episode of an angina requiring hospitalisation, which was another of the end-points in this trial. Triple counting again. Angina > stent > MI. You are not supposed to count anything but the first event, What did they do in this trial? Even after scrutinising all the available information it remains unclear to me.

Yet another problem is that it would be possible for the cardiologists seeing the patient to work out if the patient was taking vytorin, rather than simvastatin and a placebo, based on the LDL levels. Yes, the cardiologist must be informed that the patient is taking part in a clinical trial, and indeed it may well be the same cardiologist who enrolled that patient on the trial in the first place. More than likely, in fact. This leads to a significant risk of unblinding. In studies like this, neither the patient nor the person running the trial nor any clinician should know if the participant is on the drug or the placebo, which means that the study is called double blinded. But if the cardiologist knows the patient is on a trial, and knows the LDL level, they will know if the patient is taking ezetimibe or not. This will, consciously or unconsciously, change their decision-making. Another significant source of bias has been built in.

In fact, when you start to crack this trial open, you can see that we may have had double, triple counting and unblinding that will significantly affect the number of revascularisations and MIs. Yes, there were more non-fatal MIs and more coronary revascularisations in the ezetimibe group. But which caused what, and how were they counted? How complicated it all becomes. How tricky. How much bias was truly present?

I was not the only one to note this.

Dr Sanjay Kaul (Cedars Sinai Medical Center, Los Angeles, CA), who was not affiliated with the study, said the IMPROVE-IT trial 'technically' won on the primary end point, but he questions the clinical significance of the findings, noting the overall treatment effect was modest. He also points out that the difference in the composite primary end point 'was elevated to the lofty pedestal of statistical significance simply due to the large sample size, a classic example of a disconnect between statistical significance and clinical importance.'

'Are we to applaud and celebrate a 6% relative risk reduction in a quintuplet end point that is primarily driven by reductions in nonfatal end points?' asked Kaul. He added that '*it is not clear which type of MIs, spontaneous or periprocedural,* [which means it happens during the process, in this case revascularisation] *were reduced with treatment.*'[16]

Indeed, when you are looking at differences as vanishingly small as were found in this trial, even the slightest alteration in the end-points would have condemned it to failure. I calculated that five fewer events in the simvastatin arm would have led to 'statistical' failure. (Hazard ratio, 0.936 (95 per cent CI, 0.89–0.99) P=0.016. This bit of statistics is for the enlightenment of fellow geeks.)

I know that I have just spent a lot of time talking about a single clinical trial, a rather sad and disappointing trial in many ways. However, I think it is important as it highlights several issues that are key to this whole area.

It was a trial that the pharmaceutical companies clearly did not want to do. Following the disaster of ENHANCE, which itself was published nearly two years late. In fact, they had no choice other than doing IMPROVE-IT because of the failure of the ENHANCE study.

Having commenced IMPROVE-IT, they doubled recruitment, mid-trial, changed end-points and avoided setting up overall or CV mortality as the sole primary end-points. Then they created a quintuple end-point that included a non-clinical outcome (revascularisation), which is subject to bias. They also recalculated the statistics half-way through the trial, and decided not to publish the figures.

Having done all of this, they still only scraped statistical, if not clinical, significance by their fingernails Most importantly, they loudly claimed to have confirmed the LDL hypothesis by finding a non-statin drug that improved CV outcomes. The LDL hypothesis is correct. Hoorah, Wile E. Coyote can keep on thrashing wildly at the air without falling.

Even with all this, when the results of the clinical trial were presented to the Food and Drugs Administration (FDA) in the US, which seems to approve almost everything, the advisory panel rejected it.

Merck & Co should not be allowed to claim that its cholesterol-lowering drug vytorin reduces the risk of heart attacks and strokes in patients with coronary heart disease, an advisory committee to the US Food and Drug Administration concluded on Monday.

The panel evaluated data from an 18,000-patient trial known as Improve-It whose results showed that the combination treatment known as vytorin, comprising zetia and an older cholesterol-lowering drug, simvastatin, reduced the rates of heart attack, stroke and death compared with simvastatin alone.

But the panelists voted 10-5 against allowing Merck to make the claim, saying they were not convinced the benefit was clinically meaningful, especially since some patient data was missing.

'The benefit here is small,' said Dr Milton Packer, distinguished scholar in cardiovascular science at

Baylor University Medical Center. 'It is not robust. You blink and you miss it, and you wonder if you care or don't care.' [17]

Of course, ezetimibe is still being widely prescribed. Go figure.

You may ask, quite reasonably, surely there is an organisation somewhere that should be able to set and monitor trial standards.

Well, there is not. You can set up a study to measure almost anything you like. You can create your own end-points and define the statistical analyses you are going to use. Yes, there are ethics committees who can stop your study dead in the water, but only if it looks like you are doing something unethical, which normally means putting people at risk in some way.

However, ethical committees are not interested in how you approach your statistical analysis, the length of your trial, which countries you use for your study, etc. These matters will only be reviewed when you try to get your drug approved by the regulatory agencies, or when you try to publish your study.

As for publication, this relies purely on editorial and peer review. The journal editor reads the study, or more likely gets a minion to read it. There will some checks on the statistics and the methods used, etc. The manuscript will then be sent off to a couple of peer reviewers to see if they think it is okay, and that's pretty much that. Such a system is not going to have much chance of holding out against a massive international study like IMPROVE-IT, with so many key opinion leaders involved, especially opinion leaders who will be friendly with all the known peer-reviewers in the clinical area concerned.

IMPROVE-IT was a big fish for any journal to land. Not only was there massive interest in the results, which will affect its 'impact factor' in the right direction. The sponsoring company will also order tens of thousands of highly lucrative reprints, to be distributed at conferences and handed out to doctors. Turning down such a study for publication would have major financial implications for any editor.

The reality is that the publication of a major clinical trial, such as IMPROVE-IT, is pretty much guaranteed. If the *New England Journal of Medicine* (*NEJM*) doesn't publish, *The Lancet* will. If you want it published, it *will* be published. To quote Richard Horton, editor of *The Lancet*: 'Journal editors deserve their fair share of criticism too. We aid and abet the worst behaviours. Our acquiescence to the impact factor fuels an unhealthy competition to win a place in a select few journals. Our love of "significance" pollutes the literature with many a statistical fairy-tale. We reject important confirmations. Journals are not the only miscreants. Universities are in a perpetual struggle for money and talent, endpoints that foster reductive metrics, such as high-impact publication. National assessment procedures ... incentivise bad practices.'[18]

Taking another look at this issue was Marcia Angell, who edited the *NEJM*, ranked number one medical journal in the world on the dreaded 'impact factor'. She had this to say about the state of medical research, in an article from 2009, 'Drug Companies & Doctors: A Story of Corruption': 'It is simply no longer possible to believe much of the clinical research that is published, or to rely on the judgement of trusted physicians or authoritative medical guidelines. I take no pleasure in this conclusion, which I reached slowly and reluctantly over my two decades as an editor of the *New England Journal of Medicine*.'[19]

If you don't like that, try this from Richard Horton: 'The case against science is straightforward: much of the scientific literature, perhaps half, may simply be untrue. Afflicted by studies with small sample sizes, tiny effects, invalid exploratory analyses, and flagrant conflicts of interest, together with an obsession for pursuing fashionable trends of dubious importance, science has taken a turn towards darkness.'[20]

Or this, from Richard Smith, long-time editor of the *BMJ*: 'Twenty years ago this week, the statistician Doug Altman published an editorial in the *BMJ* arguing that much medical research was of poor quality and misleading. In his editorial entitled 'The Scandal of Poor Medical Research', Altman wrote that much research was seriously flawed through the use of inappropriate designs, unrepresentative samples, small sample, incorrect methods of analysis and faulty interpretation. Twenty years later I fear that things are not better, but worse ...'[21]

NEJM, Lancet, JAMA, BMJ. Four of the, if not *the* four, world's leading medical journals. Those who have edited them, or are editing them, are all of one voice. An extremely worrying voice it must be said. Much of the medical research that is published cannot be relied upon.

I wrote about much of this in a book called *Doctoring Data* and, yes, I'm repeating these quotes because they are so important – they bear repeating again and again. They should probably be tattooed on the forehead of everyone involved in medical research.

Most of the time the bias is impossible to spot. It is like a good magician's trick. The critical switch took place before you knew the trick had started. So we're not told what was *not* measured, what end-points were *not* chosen and why did they choose to study a certain population and not another. And what things did they know about the drug, and the non-target effects, that could bias the results in favour of the drug?

Information that will never be written down and never see the light of day.

You may now be thinking, where does this leave us? Can we not rely on research, published in prestigious medical journals? Well, the correct answer is, no, you cannot. What then of the regulatory agencies, the bodies that decide which drugs can be unleashed on Joe Public? The critically important ones are the FDA in the US and the European Medicines Agency (EMA). If one approves a drug, the other one will usually follow suit. The FDA carries by far the greatest clout in the world.

Both agencies look at three main things. Good manufacturing practice (GMP), which means can the company manufacture the drug free of contaminants, poisons and suchlike, and make it to a very high quality? In the bad old days, before WWII, you could stick pretty much anything you liked in a pill and sell it, and many did – and many died.

After GMP comes safety. A drug may be perfectly well manufactured, perfectly shiny and new, but can it still kill or cause other horrible things to happen? Yes, it might lower blood pressure but it also causes you to turn blue and drop dead of heart failure.

Thalidomide was the most powerful trigger for safety testing to be massively tightened up, in both Europe and the US. No one had really thought to study what might happen to the unborn child, or to try to find out if drugs had 'off-target', unwanted effects. And there was a time when you could simply whack penicillin into a few patients to see what happens, no questions asked. No chance of that today. There would be many years of safety testing first. Tests which, some now argue, may have gone a bit too far. If Ebola is killing 90 per cent of people who catch it, then you might want to reduce your safety rules a bit. The drugs can hardly do more harm than the infection. Perhaps this is a different argument for a different time.

Nowadays, before you can launch a product, you need to expose it to cultured cells, then animals, human volunteers, then more human volunteers at different doses, all the while closely monitoring what happens. Even after drugs are launched you need to keep track of what takes place in the real world, the world of elderly patients swallowing many different drugs simultaneously, etc. This is called post-marketing surveillance.

In general, manufacturing standards are now excellent and safety is good to average. Maybe not as good as you would hope. A review of drugs approved by the FDA from 2001–10 found major safety issues with nearly a third; 71 one out of 222 were withdrawn, needed a 'black box' warning, had a previously unknown adverse effect or had a safety announcement about new risks.[22]

However, the next bit causes the greatest controversy. Efficacy. Does the drug do any good? Well, you would hope, would you not, that an organisation, such as the FDA, would only approve drugs that were highly beneficial. You would also hope that some serious attempt had been made to find out how well they performed on this rather vital function. Read this statement from 2014: 'Many patients and physicians assume that the safety and effectiveness of newly approved therapeutic agents is well understood; however, the strength of the clinical trial evidence supporting approval decisions by the US Food and Drug Administration (FDA) has *not* been evaluated.'[23]

Another issue that is almost beyond belief is the regulation, review and monitoring of the centres that carry out the research. The places where the clinical trials are actually done. To be blunt about this, some countries and some researchers don't do research very well, and tend to make up the results, as highlighted in an article called 'A Clinical Trial Torpedoed by Fraud and Incompetence.'[24]

This issue was further highlighted in a *BMJ* article that looked at the evidence from trials done in more and less developed countries. It concluded that: 'Trials from less developed countries in a few cases show significantly more favourable treatment effects than trials in more developed countries and, *on average, treatment effects are more favourable in less developed countries.*' Pay your money, and get the result you want?[25]

Why are the FDA (and EMA) so lax on these critical issues? Possibly because the pharmaceutical companies, rather than Government, now provide much of the FDA's income. In 1992 the Prescription Drug User Fee Act allowed the Food and Drug Administration (FDA) to collect fees from drug manufacturers to fund the new drug approval process. To quote Marcia Angell again: 'It's time to take the Food and Drug Administration back from the drug companies ... In effect, the user fee act put the FDA on the payroll of the industry it regulates. Last year, the fees came to about $300 million, which the companies recoup many times over by getting their drugs to market faster.'[26]

Let me see, your job is to regulate an industry. However, your salary is reliant on funds from that industry. Conflict of interest is built in. And if you smugly think things are much better in Europe, think again. The problems are rampant here, too. Read 'The European Medicines Agency is still too close to industry.'[27]

Perhaps I should have warned those of a nervous disposition to look away before reading this section, as it all rather worrying. Medical research is often fatally biased and, in many cases, simply untrue. The journal editors know it, yet publish anyway. The regulatory agencies allow many unsafe medicines through, and have no idea if the processes they use to evaluate efficacy work, and most of their funding comes from the very industry they are supposed to regulate. Oh joy.

Today, we have a research and regulatory system that has grown bloated and complacent over the years, as all systems isolated from proper external review inevitably do. One could argue that it has travelled so far along this road due to the belief that scientists are less venal than the rest of humanity. Selfless individuals, only interested in finding out that most precious of all things ... the truth. Never would they fudge their results. Never would they allow themselves to be seduced by fame, and power and money. Never ...

Sorry, one can only write so much bilge. Science and research has become an industry. Publish or die, gain money from commercial sources or die. Get your papers published in high-impact journals or die. Gain funding from the pharmaceutical industry or die. And if you make the mistake of failing to find a positive outcome ... die. Pulling the strings in the background are pharmaceutical companies whose focus appears to have tightened down over the years onto one thing, and one thing alone. Money, followed by more money, and More and MORE.

What is anyone doing about it? We have a research system riven with bias, errors and very scary failings. This is well recognised by almost everyone involved in medical research and still nothing of any significance is done. Journal editors now demand that researchers disclose conflicts of interest, i.e. have they received money from the pharmaceutical industry? This must be the smallest fig leaf of the lot.

And what has happened? In many cases pharmaceutical

companies simply pay medical 'charities', or academic institutions, who then hand on the money to the researchers and opinion leaders who then claim they have no conflicts of interest because they are not paid directly by pharmaceutical companies. And we are supposed to believe this? To quote Catbert, *Mwahahahahaha!*

A couple of years ago a meeting was held to discuss such matters in London. It was reported by Richard Horton in *The Lancet*:

> 'A lot of what is published is incorrect.' I'm not allowed to say who made this remark because we were asked to observe Chatham House rules [i.e. a quote cannot can be attributed to anyone]. We were also asked not to take photographs of slides. Those who worked for government agencies pleaded that their comments especially remain unquoted, since the forthcoming UK election meant they were living in 'purdah' – a chilling state where severe restrictions on freedom of speech are placed on anyone on the government's payroll. Why the paranoid concern for secrecy and non-attribution? Because this symposium – on the reproducibility and reliability of biomedical research, held at the Wellcome Trust in London last week – touched on one of the most sensitive issues in science today: the idea that *something has gone fundamentally wrong with one of our greatest human creations.*[28] [My emphasis]

The editorial was called, 'What is medicine's 5 Sigma?' This refers to the fact that, in particle physics, significance (of any finding) is set at 5 Sigma, which means a 1 in 3.5 million chance that a finding could be purely by chance. In medical research, as mentioned before, significance is set at 1 in 20, usually written as $p < 0.05$.

Why this figure? I was told it was set by R. A. Fisher, the so-called father of classical medical statistics. He never explained, but there we are. The figure has become set in stone, unquestioned, the holy grail of statistical significance. The rock upon which research founders. A rock based on nothing at all. It just is.

Throw a dice and get two sixes in a row, that is a 1 in 36 chance. Toss a coin four times and get four heads in a row, that's 1 in 16. Add some bias to the dice, and 1 in 36 quite easily becomes 1 in 2. Perhaps evens. 'Propensity', as Karl Popper would say. You only know if bias is there, for sure, after the event – and in clinical trials that, my friends, is too late because those dice will never be thrown again. No one repeats major clinical trials – ever. It is just too damned expensive and, ironically, it would be unethical to do so.

Yes, in the most perfect twist, if a clinical trial finds that a drug has benefits in a specific condition, it would be considered unethical not to give people that drug in the future. So, if you tried to repeat IMPROVE-IT, you would be turned down on the basis that it would be unethical. Get out of that one.

Anyway, I shall leave all this for now and return to the original question. Did IMPROVE-IT prove the hypothesis that lowering LDL protects against CVD? Clearly, I am biased, as I do not believe that raised LDL causes CVD. However, I do not think it is possible to claim anything from IMPROVE-IT. It certainly did not disprove the LDL hypothesis, but you would be stretching the boundaries of reality to claim proof. Which means that, after all these years, we are still left with statins as the only agents that lower LDL and also have a discernible effect on the risk of CV mortality. Even if the effect is not large, it does exist.

Until we come to PCSK9 inhibitors.

Yes, ladies and gentlemen, we present the latest and the greatest LDL-lowering agents in history. Roll up, roll up. Gasp in awe as our PCSK9 drives LDL levels down to unimaginably low levels. Watch, as atherosclerotic plaques simply disappear into thin air. Heart disease will be banished. And for this miraculous death-defying medicine, I am not asking £50 a year. No. I am not asking £1,000 a year. No. I am asking a mere £8,000 (price may differ due to regulatory requirements of $14,000/year in the US).

A PSCK9 inhibitor, as explained, is short for proprotein convertase subtilisin/kexin type 9 inhibitor. But what does it do? It is an enzyme that breaks down the LDL receptor within the cell. Normally, after an LDL receptor locks on to an LDL molecule, and brings it into the cell, the LDL receptor itself is also broken down. If the cell needs more LDL, it must manufacture a brand spanking new receptor.

If the LDL receptor is not broken down – because the PCSK9 enzyme has been blocked – it then automatically gets stuck back out through the cell membrane to attach to a new LDL. So, more and more LDL is pulled from the bloodstream and the LDL is dragged down to very low levels indeed. (And the 'deadly' cholesterol level within cells rises to very high levels indeed – just a thought.)

At the time of writing two PCSK9 inhibitors have made it to market, evolocumab (Repatha) or alirocumab (Praluent). Note the ending -mab. This means these drugs are **M**onoclonal **A**nti**B**odies. There are many MABs, used in many different diseases, and they are – at the time of writing – the best thing since sliced bread.

In nature, antibodies are proteins produced by the body to bind to specific infective agents and suchlike, and inactivate them, also presenting them for destruction by white blood cells. They form a key part of the immune response. However, you can now manufacture synthetic (monoclonal) antibodies to bind to almost anything you like and inactivate it. PCSK9 inbibitors were designed to bind to part of the LDL receptor complex (not sure where, this is proprietary information), and stop it being broken down.

There are two other things about MABs that you need to know. First, they cannot be taken as a tablet, as they would be digested in the stomach, so they must be given by injection, rather like insulin. Second, they are usually eye-wateringly expensive. Some are nearly £100,000 per injection which, financially, is like injecting a small house or a Ferrari.

Now, I am sure when MABs first came out they were a complete ball-ache to manufacture in any quantity, and cost a fortune to make. I am equally sure that, by now, they are becoming cheap as chips. In fact, avastin, which is a MAB (bevacizumab), was expensive at first but now costs £12.13 ($15) per injection.

But why keep the price so high? Well, the main issue is that the primary competition for PCSK9s, purely with regard to LDL lowering, are statins. And since statins have lost patent protection, the price has fallen off the edge of the cliff. In the UK, simvastatin now costs about £30 a year. A high dose statin can lower LDL by around 40–50 per cent. Add in ezetimibe for another £30 a year (this is now off-patent too) and you get to 60 per cent LDL lowering for £60 a year, or thereabouts.

PCSK9s can drive LDL lower than this, but not massively. Therefore, the amount you can charge will be restricted. However, to make enough profit to cover your research and development and marketing costs, you would need to get millions of people to take a PCSK9 at £60 a year and that is a tough sell, with statins ruling the roost.

And there is another major problem. PCSK9s need to be injected once every two weeks or so. Will patients be willing to subject themselves to regular injection? Some will, many won't, some just can't. People don't like injections very much, and would resist unless absolutely necessary. You would certainly need to give some training to patients on where and how to inject, and that is a major barrier.

What to do? Imagine you oversee the global marketing for your company's PCSK9 inhibitor. You'll keep the price very high and go for a niche market. In this case that market is obvious. It is people with FH who are reckoned to be at an extremely high risk of CVD. It is a relatively straightforward argument that they absolutely must get their LDL levels as low as possible.

This can be done with a simple injection, at the very reasonable cost of £8,000 a year (terms and conditions apply). Surely this is a small price to pay? The pitiful cry of pharmaceutical company executives can be heard again. 'You must believe in the cholesterol hypothesis, children, or the hypothesis will die.'

Hold on, what is the size of this market? Is it big enough? Well, it is usually stated that 1 in 500 people have FH. The adult population of the UK is about 40 million, which means that you have potential market of 80,000 people. Being realistic, you will never get everyone with FH to take a PCSK9, but you could realistically aim to get 50 per cent, i.e. 40,000.

If a PCSK9 costs around £8,000 per year the calculation

is simple. 40,000 x £8,000 = £320 million a year. And that, ladies and gentlemen, is half-way to a blockbuster in one small country that, once upon a time, used to be part of Europe.

BLOCKBUSTER DRUGS – WHAT ARE THEY?

An extremely popular drug that generates annual sales of at least $1 billion for the company that creates it. Examples of blockbusters include Vioxx, Lipitor and Zoloft, and they are commonly used to treat common medical problems such as high cholesterol, diabetes, high blood pressure, asthma and cancer.[29]

The population of the US is six times that of the UK. This makes the US market worth, conservatively, about £2 ($3) billion a year. Drugs usually cost more in the US than anywhere else in the world, so this figure would probably be much higher. Add in the rest of Europe, Canada, Japan, China, etc., and you have a super-blockbuster, even if you only treat 50 per cent of 1 in 500 people. As you can see, there are very good reasons for keeping prices eye-wateringly high. Not least is the fact that, psychologically, the higher the price of a drug (or anything) the greater the perceived benefit.

Having said this, pharmaceutical companies still like to expand their market as much as possible, so there will be a many-pronged attack. First, a campaign to start treating children for raised cholesterol – the damage is being done early, so get them protected as soon as possible. Read this, from HEARTUK, the 'cholesterol charity': 'It is very important that all the children in the family (including brothers and sisters that are not affected) are encouraged to eat a healthy diet, to be physically active and not to start smoking. It will help if they can learn by seeing positive family role models around them. Statins are increasingly being used to treat children with Familial Hypercholesterolemia and may be started *as early as age 10.*'[30]

The next step is to move from prescribing statins to PCSK9 inhibitors. Opening the market with a thin wedge, then hammering the wedge further in is a well-established tactic.

And whilst you are working to ensure that children with FH are using PCSK9s, you can then change the definition of FH, something that has been going on for a couple of years. This 2004 article entitled 'Familial Hypercholesterolaemia' says: 'The world-wide prevalence of FH is about 1 in 500 people.'[31]

Ten years later we have an article talking about a new test for FH: 'The DNA blood test aims to spot the 1 in 500 people in the UK who have familial hypercholesterolaemia (FH), an inherited condition that greatly increases a person's heart attack risk.'[32] Before 2014 and the launch of PCSK9 inhibitors, the prevalence of FH remained steady around the world. But when we reach 2016 (after the launch of PCSK9s), a strange thing has happened. FH now affects 1 in 250 people: 'Most physicians believe that FH is rare and not often seen in practice. In fact, it is significantly more common than 1:500, the estimate made at the time that Brown and Goldstein identified the LDL receptor. Current studies suggest a prevalence of *1 in 200 to 300* people based on work in the Netherlands, Denmark, and other countries where *genetic testing* has played a significant role.'[33]

It is a matter of public record that Dr Goldberg, one of the authors of the article, receives consulting fees from **Sanofi/Regeneron** and OptumRx, research grant support from **Amarin**, Merck, ISIS, **Sanofi-Aventis**, **Regeneron, Amgen**, **Pfizer,**

Genentech/Roche, and Glaxo-Smith-Kline, and honoraria for editorial work on the Merck Manual. (I highlighted in bold the companies who were developing and/or marketing PCSK9 inhibitors at the time – Pfizer have since pulled out, as their PCSK9 was going horribly wrong.)

In 2017 the British Heart Foundation had this to say: 'FH is an inherited condition that is passed down through families and is caused by one or more faulty genes ... *Around 1 in 250* of the UK population has the condition.'[34]

Anyway, what has happened to PCSK9 inhibitors? Do they work? Well, they certainly lower LDL levels very dramatically. On that basis, they do work. They were, as you may expect, approved by the FDA in 2015, very shortly after IMPROVE-IT 'proved' that LDL lowering did improve CV outcomes. My goodness, what an amazing coincidence ...

However, unlike ezetimibe, which had no outcome data for ten years after the launch, a 'proper' outcomes study has been done. I use the term proper in its loosest possible sense. It was called the FOURIER study on Repatha (evolocumab). The first point to note about this trial is that it was designed to last at least four years, but it was stopped shortly before its second birthday. Had I the space, I would delve in some detail in to why clinical trials should not be stopped short. However, I will restrict myself to one quote on this issue: 'The tendency for truncated trials to overestimate treatment effects is particularly dangerous because their apparently compelling results often prompt publication in prominent journals, rapid dissemination in media, and speedy incorporation into practice guidelines and quality assurance initiatives.'[35] Quite.

Despite its highly premature termination, the FOURIER trial was hailed as a magnificent success and further proof of the LDL hypothesis. There were various glowing reports, including this from Medscape: 'The study, which included more than 27,000 participants with atherosclerotic CVD and already receiving statins, showed that patients who received injections of evolocumab... had a 15% reduced risk for the composite of MI, stroke, CV death, coronary revascularisation, and unstable angina hospitalisation at 22 months compared with those receiving matching placebo (P<0.001).

'For a key secondary end point—MI, stroke, or CV death—the study showed a 20% risk reduction for the evolocumab group (P<0.001).'[36]

Now, if you're paying attention, you'll notice the same quintuple end-point strategy was used as with IMPROVE-IT. It was not designed or powered to look directly at overall mortality or CV mortality. The end-points chosen were:

- CV death
- MI
- Unstable angina hospitalisation
- Stroke

And, our favourite, the end-point *du jour* ...

- Coronary revascularisation

Guess which end-point moved by the greatest amount. No prizes here, I'm afraid. Yes, coronary revascularisations. The end-point that is *not* a clinical outcome. Also, as pointed out before, if there are more revascularisations there will be more non-fatal MIs. Non-fatal MIs were, of course, the second most improved end-point.

But what were the differences in the big ones – CV and

overall mortality – the ones that really matter? Although they were not used as primary end-points for the study, they were still recorded. I suspect that, by now, you may know what is coming. Deaths from CVD:

- Total number of deaths from CVD in the Repatha group = 251
- Total number of deaths from CVD in the placebo group = 240

Yes, *11 more* people died of CVD in the Repatha/PSCK9 group. But what of the overall mortality data?

- The total number of overall deaths in the Repatha group = 444
- The total number of overall deaths in the placebo group = 426

There were *18 more* deaths in those taking Repatha/PSCK9.

Here is a drug that costs $14,000 a year and massively lowers LDL, yet has no benefit on overall or CV mortality. Whoop-,as they say, de-doo.

There is one final point I want to highlight. How facts are presented in a manner that is so misleading that they appear to say the exact opposite of what was found. So let's have a closer look at this statement: 'For a key secondary end point – MI, stroke, or CV death – the study showed a 20% risk reduction for the evolocumab group (P<0.001).'

You could be forgiven for thinking that there had been a 20 per cent reduction in CV death. Doesn't it say that? But the key word is 'or'. Taken at face value, a 20 per cent reduction in MI, stroke or CV death would be an impressive and clinically important end-point. But as you have already seen, there were more CV deaths in the Repatha group. Ho hum.

Finally, I shall attempt to gather together the evidence from the non-statin LDL-lowering trials. What have they told us? The mainstream view is that they have triumphantly confirmed the LDL hypothesis. There is, however, an alternative view; looked at together, they have triumphantly *disproved* the LDL hypothesis.

If you take all the cholesterol-lowering drug trials before statins came along, there was a significant drop in cholesterol, with no improvement in CV or overall mortality. In addition, we had the evacetrapib study – ACCELERATE – mentioned earlier, where LDL was lowered by 37 per cent with *no* effect on any CV outcome. You'd think this might have sunk the LDL hypothesis altogether. But no, it was simply treated as a paradox and then ignored. At around the same time as the failure of evacetrapib, we had the IMPROVE-IT and FOURIER trials, involving more than 45,000 participants. But neither trial showed any improvement on CV or total mortality – viewed separately or combined. It is all quite extraordinary. Abject failure presented as glorious triumph.

I sometimes feel I am simply watching a massive, psychotically deranged bluebottle fly, banging again and again against a windowpane in a desperate attempt to escape. Right next to it is an open window, but the fly just cannot see it. It will *not* move 10cm to the right. 'I will get out, I will.' In the end it is a mercy to whack it with a fly-swatter.

I use this analogy to avoid the definition of insanity as being doing the same thing again, expecting a different result. You see, I avoided that cliché rather nicely. Although, in this case, *it would be true.*

CHAPTER 10

What is a Statin?

Onwards and upwards – the statins. What *do* they do? As mentioned earlier, a statin is a drug that blocks the synthesis of cholesterol. It does this by jamming up the enzyme HMG-CoA reductase, which is required to convert 3-hydroxy-3-methylglutaryl CoA into mevalonate, which is why statins are sometimes referred to as HMG-CoA reductase inhibitors.

I have read many tales about where statins were discovered. Was it Japanese scientists looking at a substance called compactin? American scientists? Or the American Army trying to discover new poisons? Bear in mind that all drugs are poisons – if you increase the dose enough.

The story I like best is that statins were found in red yeast rice by American Army researchers looking for new ways of killing people. But they were not poisonous enough to be of much use for assassinations, so they gave the discovery to Merck to do with it what they would. Hell, I think this story might even be true.

Although they are a rubbish poison, red yeast rice plants do synthesise their own statin to ward off any animals that may find it tasty. 'Try to eat me, would you! Ingest my statin and die of low cholesterol, scum!' The statin in red yeast rice is called monacolin K. Strangely, I have never seen it referred to as a statin, even though it appears to have exactly the same chemical structure as lovastatin, the first ever statin to be launched.

This strangeness intensifies because, as far as I know, you cannot patent a chemical that you happen to stumble across otherwise there would be a mad rush to patent any chemical you found. H_2O for example. It is only possible to patent a new chemical entity that you developed all by yourself, in a laboratory. So how did Merck manage to patent monacolin K, and then call it lovastatin? Maybe there is some chemical tweak involved in converting monacolin K into lovastatin that I am unaware of. Who knows? Some questions do not appear to have any answers.

Just to make this issue clear, time for a game of spotting the difference between lovastatin and monacolin K.

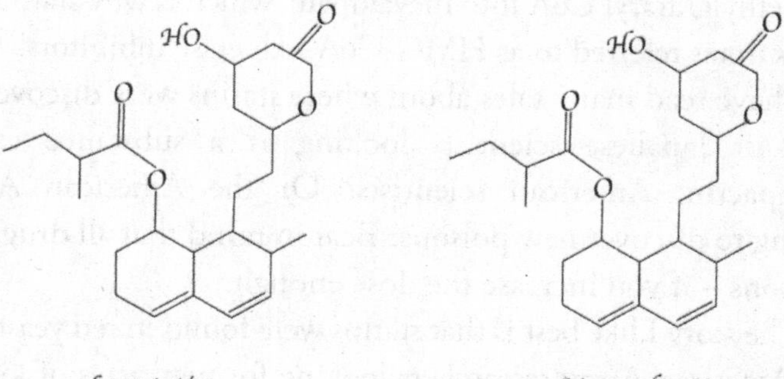

Lovastatin   Monacolin K

DIAGRAM 22

I do find it mildly amusing that some people take red yeast rice to lower their blood cholesterol levels, content that they are taking a natural substance rather than some horrible synthetic drug. Sorry guys, but the natural substance in red yeast rice is monacolin K and it is a statin, a horrible synthetic drug. Synthesised by rice, not man.

Statins first reached the healthcare market in the late 1980s. To be more precise, it was in September, in the year of our Lord 1987, that Merck launched lovastatin upon the unsuspecting world. My goodness, has it been so long. Since then, several more have popped out at regular intervals. We have, in alphabetical order:

- atorvastatin
- fluvastatin
- lovastatin
- pitavastatin
- pravastatin
- rosuvastatin
- simvastatin

Once upon a time, there was another statin called cerivastatin. It was very powerful at lowering LDL. Indeed, it was the most powerful statin of all. It was also withdrawn after causing a very high incidence of rhabdomyolysis, otherwise known as the irreversible destruction of muscle cells. When the breakdown products of the destroyed muscles hit the kidneys, this can lead to acute kidney failure and death – in a high percentage of cases. All statins can trigger rhabdomyolysis. Cerivastatin caused rather too many cases and it was hooked off stage.

Despite the failure of cerivastatin, and the occasional deaths here and there from rhabdomyolysis, statins have been *the* most profitable medications known to man. At their peak, they were bringing in around $50 billion a year in profit; over the years, I would estimate a total worldwide profit for all statins of about $1 trillion.

Things have changed dramatically in that none of the statins are protected by patent anymore, so the price has crashed. (A patent lasts for 20 years after the new chemical entity has been first registered.) The last patent to run out was for pitavastatin; at least I am pretty sure the patent has run out. Patent expiry with pharmaceuticals is a hugely complex area.

With such eye-watering profits at stake, when a generic version of their drug appears on the horizon, pharmaceutical companies tie up the courts for years arguing about manufacturing standards, formulations and licences, the exact angle of the fifth carbon hydrogen bond or whatever. Then they argue about what they are arguing about, then Heisenberg's uncertainly principle …

I can hardly blame them for throwing lawyers around and stalling for time. One extra week of patent protection for atorvastatin (Lipitor) would have been worth $189 million to Pfizer, say the chief executive's bonus for a year.

I've just realised that I haven't yet said what statins are designed to do, from a clinical perspective. However, I guess that by now everyone knows that statins lower blood cholesterol levels or, to be more accurate LDL levels. To quote from the website WebMD, chosen almost at random, from thousands of possibilities: 'Statins are a class of drugs often prescribed by doctors to help lower cholesterol levels in the blood. By lowering the levels, they help prevent heart attacks and stroke. Studies show that, in certain people, statins reduce the risk of heart attack, stroke, and even death from heart disease by about 25% to 35%. Studies also show that statins can reduce the chances of recurrent strokes or heart attacks by about 40%.'[1]

Leaving aside the slight problem that there is no such thing as a cholesterol level – they really mean LDL – this quote from WebMD is pretty much the party line on statins. They lower cholesterol and reduce the risk of death from heart disease by 25–30 per cent. Please remember these figures represent the glorious Soviet party line, and not what I happen to agree with.

PLEIOTROPIC EFFECTS

I think it is particularly important to look at the other effects of statins, as this is highly relevant to the argument that statins, where they have been shown to have a benefit, do not actually work by lowering LDL, they work in other ways.

When drugs do things in the body that they were not initially designed to do – not their primary effect – these are known as pleiotropic effects. These are not quite the same thing as side effects or drug-related adverse effects, although there is, of course, significant overlap. It is a poorly defined area.

To give a few examples of the pleiotropic actions of other drugs. Viagra was developed to treat angina. The way it worked was to open up/dilate the coronary arteries. Well, it certainly did this, but it also dilated blood vessels in the penis, which improved erections. This was discovered when army personnel who were being paid to take part in early stage clinical trials didn't hand their tablets back at the end of the trial. The researchers wondered why. The rest, as they say, is history.

Viagra is now also used to treat high blood pressure in the lungs (pulmonary hypertension). It can also be used to treat unborn babies with growth restriction in utero – it helps their lungs, hearts and blood vessels to develop properly. Furthermore, it can prevent mountain sickness (reducing blood pressure in the lungs and stopping them filling up with fluid), and it helps said mountaineers falling off mountains (joke). It also significantly lowers blood pressure in the rest of the body. In addition, it can halve the risk of dying of CVD. And yes, it is pretty good at treating angina.

If fact, if you'd been very clever, the pleiotropic effects of Viagra could easily have been worked out from first principles. With other drugs, however, they can do things that seem completely unconnected. For example, desmopressin treats bed-wetting in children and can also treat haemophilia. Go figure that one.

Aspirin is possibly the most well-known drug with widespread pleiotropic effects. It was first used to treat fever, aches and pains. It was then found to be effective in the treatment of myocardial infarction, then in the long-term prevention of CVD. Now, it is being used to reduce the risk of cancer.

Perhaps one of the most interesting examples is thalidomide. It was launched as a drug to treat insomnia and morning sickness, but was then found to lead to terrible malformations in unborn children and was withdrawn from the market. The very name thalidomide still sends shivers down the spine. However, it has been reborn. It now used to treat certain types of cancer, under a different name. It can also be prescribed for leprosy, HIV, lupus and Crohn's disease.

As with Viagra, once you knew more about how thalidomide works, you could have worked out the benefits and harms it would cause. I didn't, but someone else did. Many things are obvious when they are pointed out. Fascinatingly, the benefits and harms of thalidomide and Viagra are closely linked through a single chemical, namely nitric oxide (NO). Viagra stimulates it, thalidomide blocks it.

NO is a critical substance for CV health. Perhaps *the* critical substance. It is both produced by, and protects, the endothelium. It causes the smooth muscle in blood vessels to relax, thus opening arteries and preventing angina attacks. It also lowers blood pressure, stimulates the growth of new blood vessels (collaterals) in the heart and drives the production of endothelial progenitor cells (EPCs) in the bone marrow. (EPCs repair any damaged areas of endothelium.)

Furthermore, it is the most potent anticoagulant in nature. Not bad for one of the simplest chemicals there is: one nitrogen atom, one oxygen atom and one free electron, ready and willing to react with anything that moves. It shouldn't really exist in the body for more than a trillionth of a second, and most scientists believed it could not. But it does, and it can be found all over the place, doing a million different things.

I think it is true to say that NO is the single most vital substance for CV health there is. As for thalidomide, it reduces NO synthesis but in the developing baby NO is actually required to stimulate blood vessel growth. Without blood vessels growing properly the limbs cannot get blood supply, so they either do not develop or become terribly shortened.

Fascinatingly, if you give thalidomide to pregnant animals, then give other drugs to stimulate NO synthesis, e.g. Viagra, you can virtually eliminate birth defects.[2] Which leads on to the reason why thalidomide works in cancer treatment. It is because, as cancers increase in size, they need their own blood supply to feed themselves, so they create their own blood vessels (angiogenesis). If you stop angiogenesis, cancer growth will be seriously inhibited, and this is the mechanism of the action of thalidomide. In one of those strange twists of nature, the same mechanism that causes birth defects also inhibits cancer growth. Who'd have guessed?

The interconnected tales of Viagra and thalidomide highlight that fact that it is almost impossible to over-emphasise the importance of NO in vascular health. Anything which improves NO synthesis *will* be highly beneficial and will reduce the risk of dying of CVD. On the other hand, anything that reduces NO synthesis *will* cause harm and increase the risk of CVD. I have found no contradictions to these statements, anywhere, in any study. Ever. Which takes us back to statins because the primary pleiotropic effect of statins is that they, too, increase NO synthesis in endothelial cells.[3] As a direct result of this:

- They lower blood pressure[4]
- They are an anticoagulant, similar in effect to aspirin[5]
- They increase the production of cells in the bone marrow that protect the lining of the arteries.

One would imagine these finding may have led to a lively debate about whether the benefits of statins on CVD are due to their effect on LDL lowering, or their effect on NO synthesis. I would be happy to have this debate anywhere, with anyone. Unfortunately, it is difficult to have a debate in an empty room.

Having said this, the pleiotropic effect of statins is something that does emerge from the depths from time to time. This report entitled 'The Potential Relevance of the Multiple Lipid-Independent (Pleiotropic) Effects of Statins in the Management of Acute Coronary Syndromes' says: 'Statins possess multiple beneficial effects that are independent of low-density-lipoprotein cholesterol (LDL-C) lowering and that have favorable effects on inflammation, *the endothelium, and the coagulation cascade.*'[6]

My own view is that any benefits of statins on CVD can be fully, indeed far better, explained by their beneficial impact on NO synthesis. LDL lowering is just an unfortunate adverse effect that it would be nice to remove.

THE STATIN TRIALS

They have been hailed as the wonder drugs, scattering down fantastic benefits upon a grateful public, with no adverse effect at all. But how effective are statins? This can be difficult to discuss or explain. I have already run through some of the games that are played in clinical studies. However, they pale into insignificance when you try to explain the next bit. How the data is unleashed on an unsuspecting world.

You may think that there is an agreed way to present the findings of a clinical study. Of course, there is not. It is a complete, bloody mess. Here are a few of the measures that are used:

- Increase in median survival
- Lives saved
- Odds ratio (OR)
- Relative risk (RR)
- Absolute risk (AR)
- Hazard ratio (HR)
- Kaplan-Meier survival curve
- Reduction in Mean Survival Time (RMST)
- Number needed to treat (NNT)

Most doctors have no idea what any of these things really mean and they don't ask, partly for fear of sounding stupid. Instead, they get shown attractive graphs that make the drugs seem shiny, brand new and unbelievably effective by mostly young, charming pharmaceutical company reps chirruping, 'And, if I may say so, are you not looking very handsome and/ or attractive today doctor?' How could anyone not prescribe this wondrous medication?

The primary method used to hype the benefit of any drug is to talk about relative risk. To explain this in as few words as I can possibly manage – the absolute risk represents the underlying risk of something unpleasant happening to you. For example, dying or being seriously injured in a car crash or while cycling, riding a motorbike or even walking.[7]

DEATHS PER BILLION MILES TRAVELLED		
Mode of transport	Deaths	Serious Injuries
Car driver	3	26
Pedestrian	42	542
Pedal cyclist	35	1035
Motorcycle rider	122	1868

Now, if you did something that doubled the risk of a car driver dying every billion miles, that would increase the absolute number of deaths by three. If you doubled the risk for motorbike riders, that would increase the absolute number of deaths by 122. The relative increase in death is, in both cases, 100 per cent. However, the absolute increase is 3 v 122, or a difference of 4,000 per cent.

As you can see, increasing the relative risk by 100 per cent means something completely different if the underlying (absolute) risks were widely separated to start with. Equally, decreasing the relative risk means something completely different, depending on the underlying absolute risk.

For example, a 66 per cent reduction in the relative risk of dying, for car drivers, would mean two fewer deaths per billion miles travelled. Reducing the risk of death by 66 per cent for motorbike riders would mean 80 fewer deaths. Whilst the relative reduction is the same, there is a massive different in absolute risk reduction.

In a clinical study, as with road deaths, the critical figure is the absolute risk reduction. Indeed, the relative risk reduction is completely meaningless if you do not know the absolute risk to start with. These figures are often buried very deeply. So let's now move onto some figures that have been presented from the clinical trials themselves. Pfizer, in US adverts for Lipitor (atorvastatin), stated that: 'Lipitor reduces risk of heart attack by 36%.'[8] Now, what do you think that means? Clearly, this figure of 36 per cent is a relative risk reduction and will include all forms of heart attack, fatal and non-fatal.

If you drill down into the figures, the *absolute* difference in the number of heart attacks was 1.1 per cent. Or, to put it another way, 98.9 per cent of those taking the drug did not benefit. There is also no mention of the time scale. Reducing the number of heart attacks by 1.1 per cent would be quite impressive if this happened within three months, but rather less impressive over five years, as this would be a reduction of 0.27 cent per year.

So, a 36 per cent reduction in the risk of a heart attack turns out to be a 0.27 per cent absolute risk reduction in heart attacks, per year. And there's no attempt to make it clear if they were talking about fatal, non-fatal or peri-procedural heart attacks. Does this now sound a little less impressive?

On the other hand, when it comes to adverse effects, absolute risk is the preferred measure of the pharmaceutical companies. If 2 out of 100 people suffer a rash taking a statin, compared with 1 in 100 taking placebo, this is not presented as a 100 per cent increase in this adverse effect. Of course not. It is presented as a 1 per cent increase. Naughty, naughty.

How do they get away with using relative risk to hype benefits, and absolute risk to downplay harm? Because, once again, there is no system in place to stop it. Only the golden rule applies here. He who has the gold makes the rules.

Another rule of statin trials, in fact of all such trials, is to look for what is *not* said. By far the most significant outcome at the end of a trial is dead or alive. There is not much point in taking a drug to reduce death from a heart attack if it increases the risk of death from kidney failure by the same amount, unless you particularly fear dying of a heart attack. Dead is dead.

Therefore, if you see a triumphal press release talking about fantastic benefits on this or that outcome, always look for overall mortality. If it is not mentioned, it did not change. Or, in some cases, it got worse, which is what happened with PCSK9s. And it's the same for any other outcome, e.g. CV mortality. If it is not mentioned, there is a reason why. Either it did not change or it got worse.

For the uninitiated, though, how can you hack your way through such cleverly manipulated hype? I have spent many years looking at clinical trials and I think I know most of the games that are played. However, I am acutely aware that for most people this is unfamiliar and difficult, and requires a lot of adding up. It is why I wrote *Doctoring Data*, and I do not want to go over that again in such detail. My brain nearly blew up writing it. So, I am going to try and make this as pain free as possible. Leaving aside adverse effects for the moment – muscle aches and pain, etc. – there are only two points you need to know from the statin trials.

The first is how much longer will you live for if you take a statin? And that's not the same thing as an improvement in overall mortality. Second, how many nasty but not fatal conditions did statins prevent, e.g. non-fatal strokes and non-fatal heart attacks.

In cancer trials the key outcome measure is usually the increase in median survival, which can be roughly translated as 'how much longer can you expect to live if you take this drug?' I can see medical statisticians exploding on the horizon as I make that statement. But I shall stick with it. It is close enough.

In CV trials you are never given this information. Ever. In fact, I am always slightly amazed that patients don't ask: 'If I take these statins, how much longer will I live, doc?' In cancer treatment this, or something very similar, is *the* number one question. I find it hard to understand why people taking statins are so completely uninterested in improved lifespan. Perhaps the bogus 36 per cent figure draws a line under that conversation. More likely, I suppose, a diagnosis of cancer carries with it the inevitable subtext of imminent death, in a way that being told you have heart disease does not.

There are also statistical reasons why it is more difficult to work out how much longer you will live if you take a statin. However, the maths can be done, and has been. But first a bit of context. Make a cup of coffee, stretch and relax, and breathe.

Most statins trials have lasted about five years. The critical ones have looked at statin v placebo, otherwise known as placebo-controlled studies. They have generally been split into primary and secondary prevention trials:

- A primary prevention trial looks at people with no previously diagnosed CVD (low risk)
- A secondary prevention trials looks at people who already have diagnosed CVD (high risk)

In primary prevention, you are trying to stop a first CV event, usually a stroke or heart attack. In secondary prevention you are trying to stop a second CV event. The underlying risk in secondary prevention studies is, by their nature, considerably higher than in primary prevention studies.

At the end of the trial, the plan is that more people will be alive after taking statins than the placebo, something that has even occurred in one or two of the trials. I am going to use one of them as an example. The Heart Protection Study (HPS).

The results were massively hyped. This trial may even have been a 'game changer'. Here are a couple of quotes from the original HPS press release, now, strangely, removed from the internet. 'LIFE-SAVER: World's largest cholesterol lowering trial reveals massive benefits for high risk patients ... Statins are the new aspirin.' It finished: In this trial ten thousand people were put on a statin. If now, an extra 10 million high-risk people worldwide go onto statin treatment *this would save about 50,000 lives each year – that's a thousand a week.*'

A thousand lives saved ... Each week.

You may be slightly less impressed to know that the absolute reduction in overall mortality in HPS was 1.8 per cent over five years, Or 0.36 per cent per year. Which, if you treat ten million people, is 36,000 per year not 50,000. Personally, I don't think 36,000 is 'about 50,000' but that is not the main issue here.

You could, of course, present this finding in a rather more low-key fashion. If you treated 200 people for a year there would be no benefit for 199. Only one extra person would still be alive. Yes, the same facts can sound very different depending on how you choose to present them. (Ten million divided by 50,000 is 200, BTW.)

But it doesn't stop here, oh no. There is another question that needs to be asked, one that is never asked. How much longer, on average, would that 1 person in 200 be expected to live? One thing for sure, it ain't going to be forever. Not even the most ardent statin advocate has claimed that statins confer immortality. Or to put this another way, just because 1.8 per cent extra people are alive at the end of five years, that does not mean that their lives have been 'saved'. This is a silly and unscientific claim to make. You can only prolong life, not banish death.

What really matters, therefore, is a combination of two things.

- How many more people were alive at the end of trial?
- How much longer were those people then likely to live?

In truth, you cannot work this out for a single person. It is impossible for any doctor to tell any specific patient, 'Yes, *you* will be the 1 in 200 whose life will be prolonged.' You can only use averages. (For the pedants amongst us, you cannot use the median, it does not exist in CV trials.)

This is the weakness of the average figure here. No one can

be average here. You cannot be 1/200th alive. You will either be alive or dead and, if you are one of the lucky ones, your gain in life expectancy will be greater than the average figure. I hope that makes sense.

Having got that out of the way. What then is the average increase in life expectancy from taking a statin in both primary and secondary prevention over around five years?

- Average increase in life expectancy in primary prevention was 3.2 days
- Average increase in life expectancy in secondary prevention was 4.1 days[9]

So, in answer to the question that no one ever asks – 'If I take these statins for five years, how much longer am I likely to live, doc?' – I can reply, 'On average, between three and four days.'

Yes, figures are funny old things. A 36 per cent reduction in heart attacks sounds fantastically impressive. Equally, saving 1,000 lives a week seems like something we absolutely must do. The reality is rather more prosaic. Take a statin for five years and live an extra four days – max.

HOW MANY SERIOUS ADVERSE EVENTS WILL STATINS DELAY?

Statin supporters regularly make the argument that, yes statins may not have demonstrated any great benefits on overall mortality. In many trials, no benefit at all, but they still prevent very unpleasant serious events. So, you cannot just look at the impact on mortality. Statins have other major benefits.

This is a reasonable argument. A non-fatal stroke can leave

you paralysed, unable to talk or feed yourself. A non-fatal MI can leave you with serious heart failure, unable to walk more than a few steps, breathless, full of fluid and struggling to breathe when lying down. These are most definitely things to be avoided, if possible.

On the other hand, a minor stroke, sometimes called a transient ischaemic attack, can last half an hour and leave the person completely unimpaired. Equally, a non-fatal MI, during say a revascularisation procedure, could pass unnoticed by the patient, only picked up by a fleeting rise in cardiac (heart) enzymes.

In my opinion, if you are counting the number of CV events, you really need to define what you are counting. The severe, debilitating and permanent, or the mild and transient with no lasting impairment? Of course, this is never done. A stroke is a stroke, a heart attack is a heart attack. No differentiation is allowed. How mad is that? Of course, this is not mad, there is a reason for it, a reason that does not take much guessing at.

In addition, during a clinical trial, many other things can happen to you that are not strokes or heart attacks. You could be admitted to hospital with angina, have a pulmonary embolus, develop kidney failure or get hit by a bus. These would all be considered serious adverse events (SAEs), and they should all be counted, both for those taking the statin and the placebo. Why? Because if statins reduce the risk of strokes and heart disease only to increase the risk of developing kidney failure, liver failure or getting hit by a bus, then you have simply exchanged one nasty thing for another. In which case, any benefit on CV events effectively disappears.

So, what are the rates of SAEs in the statin trials. Here we find ourselves struggling. All the data on the statin trials have been gathered together by an organisation in Oxford, known as the Cholesterol Treatment Trialists Unit (CTT), under the guidance of Professor Sir Rory Collins. And ... and they won't let anyone see their data. It is a secret. No, I am not making this up. As their own website says: 'Individual patient data from each contributing trial have been provided to the CTT Collaboration on the understanding that they would be used only for the purpose of the CTT meta-analyses and *would not be released to others.*'[10]

You would think that information about adverse effects, and serious adverse events, would be the sort of thing that absolutely cannot be kept secret, for the good of humanity. But it is. I don't see anyone marching on the streets about this, but they should be.

Despite this rather significant problem, another group did try to analyse the SAEs in statin trials, using the available published data, otherwise known as the data not kept secret by the CTT. This group was the Cochrane Collaboration, which is just about the only unbiased group of researchers in the world, with no financial ties to anyone. Whilst no one is perfect, they are as close to the perfect researchers as you will find. As they themselves say: 'The Cochrane Collaboration is *regarded as the gold standard of systematic reviews.* One of its guiding principles is avoiding unnecessary duplication: any independent reviewer following the proper methodology would include the same trials, extract the same data and come to the same interpretation and conclusions. The review is then updated as new trials are published.'[11]

The Cochrane Collaboration looked at SAEs in primary prevention trials and asked: 'How can CHD SAEs decrease, but not total SAEs?' In English. How can non-fatal strokes and heart attacks be reduced by statins, with no overall reduction in SAEs? Well, you know the answer to this question, and the Cochrane Collaboration came to the same conclusion: 'All CHD events are SAEs and are counted in both categories. Therefore, a reduction in major CHD SAEs should be reflected in a reduction in total SAEs. The fact that it is not suggests that other SAEs are increased by statins negating the reduction in CHD SAEs in this population. *A limitation of our analysis is that we could not get total SAE data from all the included RCTs.* However, we are confident that the data from the 6 missing RCTs would not change the results, because they represent only 41.2% of the total population and include ALLHAT-LLT, where one would not expect a reduction in total SAEs; in that trial there was no effect on mortality or cardiovascular SAEs.'[12]

Yes, even the mighty Cochrane Collaboration cannot prise the data from the lair of the CTT. However, they did find that the total SAEs were unchanged by statins. To put this another way, statins caused as many serious adverse events as they prevented (delayed). Or, to put it another way, they didn't do any bloody good.

So, bringing this together, what do we know about statins?

- They can increase life expectancy for about three to four days for every five years of treatment
- They have no benefit on SAEs

And the reality may be even worse than that. The vanishingly small benefits in the published studies may not even exist at all. Let me take you back to 2005, or maybe 1997. Both are key, as I'll explain.

For many years it was possible to set up and run a clinical

study without having to inform anyone you were even doing it. There was also no requirement to tell anyone what clinical outcomes you were looking at, and why. In addition, you did not need to show anyone the statistical analyses you were using or anything much else for that matter. At worst, you could carry out a large clinical trial, and if it was negative you could simply bury it, never to be seen again. Or you could adjust the end-points and outcomes that you claimed you were seeking, after the study was finished, Basically, you could do pretty much anything you liked. It was the Wild West, where lawmen were few and far between.

However, in 1997 US law mandated the creation of a clinical trial registry (clinical trials.gov). From the year 2000 researchers were required to record their trial methods and outcome measures *before* collecting data. The industry managed to sidestep this requirement at first. I'm not sure how, this seems unclear. Perhaps by not registering in the US. But for other researchers in the US, the effect on clinical trials was immediate and dramatic, and the results should worry us all. A study published in *Nature* looked at 55 large trials testing heart disease treatments (not necessarily industry sponsored). What they found was the following:[13]

- 57 cent of those studies published before 2000 reported positive effects from the treatments
- 8 per cent in studies that were conducted after 2000 reported positive effects from the treatments

This was reported in the article as 'Registered clinical trials make positive findings vanish.' In relative terms, there was an 86 per cent reduction in positive studies. Things then tightened up even more. In 2005 the European Union joined the US to create New Regulatory Rules for Clinical Trials, which stated that 'Every report on a clinical trial must now show verification of registration of that trial in a recognised database.' Medical journal editors got together to state that they wouldn't publish anything not registered in this way, something that doesn't happen as consistently as you might hope.

What has been the effect? Well, prior to 2005 almost every single major statin trial, bar ALLHAT-LLP, was positive. Since 2005 the benefits of statins vs placebo have dried up, as highlighted in the journal article 'Cholesterol confusion and statin controversy'. 'Curiously, statin trials conducted after 2005 have failed to demonstrate a consistent mortality benefit.'[14] What does this mean? In effect, we cannot really trust the results of any clinical trial done before 2005. It also means that we do not even know what trials were done before 2005. Negative results could simply have been buried. Evidence that this did happen comes from a review of anti-depressant drugs.

There was a major scandal that involved trial data being deliberately withheld from a study, which showed that adolescents were more likely to commit suicide if they took an SSRI (the most widely prescribed type of antidepressant). It was headline news for a while, and GSK were fined $3 billion for their involvement. Using the freedom of information act, a group of researchers then managed to find both the published and unpublished clinical trials on SSRIs. They also re-analysed the published data at the same time. What they found was that there have been:

- 38 positive trials (all but one was published)

- 36 studies deemed to be negative. Of these, only three were published as negative, 22 were simply not published and 11 studies were published as positive, when they were not.[15]

Putting this another way, if an SSRI trial was positive it was published; if it was negative the data was manipulated to make it look positive or it was buried. So ...

Yes, you can believe that statins work if you want. You can believe that they cause no adverse effects, if that helps you to sleep at night. You can believe that the grown-ups are in charge, and are all working tirelessly to ensure that ineffective and potentially damaging drugs are not waved through by committees who are all hopelessly financially conflicted. Yes, indeedy, believe that if you want.

I shall sign off here by quoting Ben Goldacre on the effect of the 2005 guidelines.

Many people think this problem has already been solved. The medical journals said they weren't going to publish trials that hadn't been registered and there were steps by the US government to require it ...

But unfortunately, there was no routine public audit and when one was finally done, many years after this rule came into play, we discovered that academic journal editors had not kept that promise.

A study found that that half of all trials published in the top ten journals in the big five fields of medicine weren't properly registered and many were not registered at all – and that's only the one's we know about.[16]

CHAPTER 11

The Downside
of Statins

I was at a doctors' all-day educational meeting recently, where various presentations were made about the latest, best treatments. One thing that stood out for me was a discussion on heart disease treatment. The presenter had coined the phrase 'heart hug' as in, 'Have you done everything possible to look after the patient's heart?' In this case it was diabetes.

Two drugs were then mentioned as providing a special heart hug. The first was metformin, the second was, of course, a statin. Give your heart a hug with a statin. Yes, when we were five.

James James
Morrison Morrison
Weatherby George Dupree
Took great
Care of his Mother,

Though he was only three.
James James said to his Mother,
'Mother,' he said, said he;
'You must never go down
To the end of the town,
If you don't go down with me.'
(From A. A. Milne's 'Disobedience', but please replace
'James' with 'statin'.)

There is nothing more powerful in life than creating an emotional bond with something. Statins have moved from being an HMG Co-A reductase inhibitor, a rather dry and scientific enzyme inhibitor, to your friend, your mummy and daddy, to tuck you in at night.

Statins, you see, do not merely lower cholesterol they give your heart a hug. I realised then that criticism of statins had become virtually impossible, those lovey-fluffy heart-hugging friends of humanity. Attacking statins would be like machine-gunning bunny rabbits.

But machine-gun bunny rabbits I shall. Statins might look like bunny rabbits but at night, when the moon is full, they turn into flesh-eating were-rabbits that'll rip your throat out. I have a book, sitting on my bookshelf, entitled *Statins Toxic Side Effects* where the author, David Evans, gathered together 500 scientific research papers outlining the wide range of damage that statins can do.

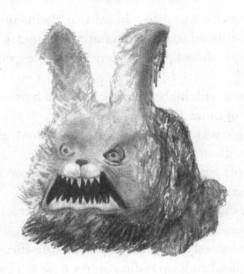

THE TRUE FACE OF STATINS – 'I'LL GIVE YOUR HEART A HUG MWAHAHAHAHAHAHAHA!'

This is not Micky Mouse stuff. Opening pages 80–1, at random, there are short summaries of studies from: *The Journal of the American Academy of Dermatology*, *Cancer*, *Cancer Epidemiology*, and *Clinical Endocrinology*, all-well respected medical journals.

The papers are entitled, in turn:

- 'Long term statin use increases the risk of basal cell carcinoma by 30%'
- 'Statin users have a 14% increased risk of melanoma'
- 'Statin users have a 25% increased risk of developing Merkel cell carcinoma'
- 'The association between statins and thyroid cancer'

Now, you have probably heard that statins protect against cancer. The disconnect between statin headlines in newspapers, and reality, is almost perfect. Here is how the game works.

- People with higher cholesterol levels have a lower risk of cancer[1]
- People with higher cholesterol levels have generally been given statins
- People given statins are found to have lower levels of cancer than people not given statins
- It is then claimed that statins protect against cancer
- Almost everyone believes this is a true effect
- My head ends up resting on my desk as I lose the will to live

Do statins cause cancer? Yes, I believe they do. Do they cause a greatly increased risk of cancer? No, I do not believe so. For example, the incidence of melanoma in the UK is 32 new cases per 100,000 people per year. A 14 per cent increase would result in around 1 extra case per 100,000 per year – not everyone takes statins.

Now, 80 per cent of melanomas are found and treated. Ergo, statins could (assuming that the study mentioned is correct) lead to one-quarter of an extra death from melanoma per 100,000 people per year. Of course, you can present this another way. This would be about 100 extra deaths per year in the UK, and 600 in the US, which does sound rather more serious. The headline writes itself: 'Statins Kill Hundreds with Cancer Worldwide Every Year' – shock horror.

But there is another important issue at play here. Namely,

who is going to spot such an increase? If statins do increase the risk of melanoma by 14 per cent, it will pass unnoticed. A single doctor will never see 100,000 patients in their lifetime. Even if they did, they would hardly notice one extra fatality from melanoma in a patient taking statins. And even if they were alerted, what could or would they do about it?

Equally, even in a clinical trial studying 10,000 patients over five years, many things will be missed. The absolute numbers are just too small. When clinical trials do not raise the alarm, this does not mean there are not major and significant problems. Indeed, we know that highly significant and damaging effects of statins have been completely missed. Let's look at cerivastatin. In 1997 this was one of the last of the statins to be unleashed on the public. It was, I think, the most potent at reducing LDL levels.

This is what was written about it in 1998 in a report called 'Cerivastatin in primary hyperlipidemia – a multicenter analysis of efficacy and safety': 'Cerivastatin is generally well tolerated and adverse events have usually been mild and transient. The overall incidence and nature of adverse events reported with cerivastatin in clinical trials was similar to that of placebo.'[2]

And this is what was said about it, slightly later, in 1998: 'The good tolerability of cerivastatin was reflected in a low rate of premature withdrawal from treatment, below or comparable to that of placebo-treatment. The pooled efficacy and safety analyses have shown that at 1% of the doses of other statins, cerivastatin is a safe, well-tolerated, and highly effective HMG-CoA reductase inhibitor.'[3]

And in 2001: 'Cerivastatin was recently withdrawn from the market because of 52 deaths attributed to drug-related rhabdomyolysis that lead to kidney failure. Rhabdomyolysis was 10 times more common with cerivastatin than the other five approved statins.'[4]

Rhabdomyolysis, as mentioned before, is a catastrophic breakdown of muscle cells, and the breakdown products then travel to the kidneys leading to death. Rhabdomyolysis has been seen with all statins, at a low(ish) level. However, the 1,000 per cent increase with cerivastatin was apparently not picked up in any clinical trial. Do you feel safe now?

Another example that highlights the inability of clinical trials to pick up dangerous problems is that statins were studied in many clinical trials, for over 30 years, before it was finally noticed they cause diabetes. This was picked in the JUPITER trial in 2008.[5] Now that people have been made aware of the connection, the increased risk of diabetes is thought to be very nearly 50 per cent (perhaps as high as 80 per cent). In fact, in a long-term study the risk of diabetes was found to increase by 363 per cent.[6]

Yet was this never noticed before? Ever?[7]

Of course, with diabetes you could argue that *it* was more difficult to disentangle than with rhabdomyolysis. Rhabdomyolysis is almost never seen, unless you take a statin, so the connection with the drug can be made very quickly, a bit like thalidomide and very specific birth deformities.

However, diabetes is a different matter. Millions of people are put on statins, millions of people have diabetes. However, not everyone with diabetes takes a statin, not by any manner of means. Could any individual doctor make the connection in an individual patient? No, or at least they would have to be looking for it – and why would they do that? Everyone thinks it is everyone else's job to do that.

Equally, if you saw a patient with a motor neurone disease who was taking statins, would you make a connection? No, you would not. However, the WHO believe they may have heard a signal amongst the noise.[8] Yes, that's right, motor neurone disease. One of the most awful diseases you can suffer from.

However, my overriding concern about statins is that they cause a crushing burden of adverse effects that are insidious, often coming on slowly, often mimicking the impact of ageing. So much so that they are simply written off as, 'What do you expect, you are getting older?' Fatigue, memory problems, muscle pain, joint pain.

I watched my father-in-law reach the state where he literally could not stand unaided, let alone walk more than 10 yards. This didn't happen overnight, it didn't even happen in the first two or three years of taking statins. It was slow, insidious and difficult to put your finger on. When he came off statins, reluctantly, fearfully, he regained the ability to get out of a chair and walk upstairs and his mood improved greatly.

I have seen the same thing with many patients, one elderly woman who literally rose from her bed and walked again. A woman transformed from a demented, immobile, 'end of life' case to a normal person again. The nurses in the unit were stunned by her complete transformation. Once you have seen that happen, your view on the impact of statins on the human body undergoes something of a conversion.

Some patients have been so terrified of stopping their statins, even those demonstrating barn door adverse effects, that they would not, indeed do not, stop. Others who did stop found that it was like removing a rucksack full of bricks and the fuzz disappeared from their brains. Bernard Lown, a famous cardiologist, free-thinker and hero of mine described his experience on statins:

An astounding lesson of my many decades of medical practice was the commonality of adverse drug reactions. Strange that I myself over several years was a victim. I developed a neuropathy, consisting of shooting, stinging, sharp electric shocks radiating from buttocks to toes, waking me nearly nightly from sound sleep. Visits to doctors and neurologists were unavailing. I was on no new medications and had been taking the same pills for more than a decade.

I began to believe that drugs were implicated. The likeliest was a statin drug, the ever-popular Lipitor. Based on my cholesterol level I had reduced it to only three times weekly. Every physician I had visited dismissed my suggestion. Statins had a low-risk profile and almost never induced neuropathic pains. I had been taking it over many years without symptoms and in a minuscule dose.

Though 'irrational,' I stopped Lipitor. Within three days the symptoms disappeared. For the first time in several years I slept through the night without discomfort. It seemed miraculous. Ever the skeptic scientist, I restarted the Lipitor. Within three days, the very same symptoms recurred, only to disappear again on drug cessation.[9]

However, at this point we reach another almost perfect disconnect between patient-reported adverse effects and what the experts tell us. The experts have now informed us, in all seriousness, that statins do not cause any adverse effects, at all. Not one. Any reported adverse reaction is due to the nocebo effect. (This the opposite of the placebo effect; you imagine aches and pains, etc., because you believe you are going to suffer them from taking the drug. Not because they are real.)

Now I am certain that some people do imagine adverse effects, to a certain extent. However, to dismiss all adverse effects is just the most absolute paternalistic nonsense. I wrote a blog about this, starting: 'Some of you may have noted that researchers have now decided that statins do not have any side effects at all. To be pedantic, the correct term is not side effects but "drug-related adverse events". A side effect can be positive, or negative.'

To prove that statins cause no adverse events, a paper was published in *The Lancet* entitled: 'Adverse events associated with unblinded, but not with blinded, statin therapy in the Anglo-Scandinavian Cardiac Outcomes Trial – Lipid-Lowering Arm (ASCOT-LLA): a randomised double-blind placebo-controlled trial and its non-randomised non-blind extension phase.' A virtually impenetrable title that could mean almost anything. But the key message can be found here: 'These analyses illustrate the so-called nocebo effect, with an excess rate of muscle-related AE (adverse event) reports only when patients and their doctors were aware that statin therapy was being used and not when its use was blinded. These results will help assure both physicians and patients that most AEs associated with statins are not causally related to use of the drug and should help counter the adverse effect on public health of exaggerated claims about statin-related side-effects.'

Stripping aside the horrible dead science speak, I shall translate. 'You only think you are having an adverse effect from taking a statin, the reality is that you have been fooled into thinking this. You are not. So stop whinging, you pathetic worm. By the way, anyone who criticises statins should probably be thrown into jail.' A sentiment later echoed by Steven Nissen in his jolly editorial entitled 'Statin Denialism, A Deadly Internet-Driven Cult'.[10]

I have met some people who appear to suffer no problems at all from taking statins and are very happy to continue taking them. I have met more whose obvious and clear-cut adverse effects have been angrily dismissed by their doctor. I have met even more who have been basically told: 'Well, muscle pain is a small price to pay to avoid dying of a heart attack.'

I have met *even* more who have just stopped taking statins, but have not informed their doctor because they are afraid of being scolded. The shelves of bathroom cabinets around the world must groan under the weight of unopened packets of statins. If you could turn statins into biofuel, the energy supplies of the world could easily be met.

The largest study on why people stopped taking statins was done in the US. It was found that 'More than six in ten respondents (62%) said they discontinued their statin due to side effects, with the secondary factor (17%) being medication cost. Only 12% of respondents cited lack of efficacy in cholesterol management as a reason for stopping their medication. On average, respondents who experienced side effects due to their statin stopped after trying two different statins.

'Three out of ten respondents experienced side effects of muscle pain and/or weakness, and 34% stopped taking their statin because of these side effects without consulting with their doctor.'[11]

In fact, after a year, nearly three-quarters of people simply stopped taking statins, mostly due to adverse effects. In contrast, the *Lancet* paper claimed to have found an increase of 0.26 per cent in statin-reported adverse effects when people knew they were taking statins. They then extrapolated this utterly minuscule figure to state that this accounts for all reported adverse effects. Nonsense beyond nonsense. Their figures don't even remotely add up, and all efforts to gain further information from the authors have been met by silence.

However, doctors now have the perfect excuse to dismiss all reported adverse effects because a study in *The Lancet*, no less, has told them that statins cause no problems at all. It is all in your mind. I presume this means that all adverse effects, of all drugs, can also be dismissed in the same way. It certainly makes the job of being a doctor much easier. 'No, you are now perfectly well and if you don't think you feel any better it is because of the nocebo effect. So please shut up and stop complaining. Next patient, *please*!'

The reality with statins is that they cause a heavy burden of adverse effects. Most of them are far from unique to statins and are quite common general complaints in the first place. Muscle pain, forgetfulness, brain fog, abdominal discomfort, lack of energy, depression, cataracts and aggression, all this is very common. Unfortunately, they are all things that many people suffer from without taking statins. Therefore, an increase in symptoms is easily dismissed.

What about the rare but highly serious effects? Well, what is clear is that you cannot trust that they will be picked up in the clinical trials. The link between cerivastatin and rhabdomyolysis was missed, and the fact that statins cause diabetes passed unnoticed for over thirty years. What else was missed? Who knows? Here are six more that worry me:

- Heart failure
- Idiopathic pulmonary fibrosis
- Degenerative neurological diseases
- MS
- Parkinson's
- Alzheimer's

And, just to finish, here's a quote on statins and Parkinson's: 'Statin use was associated with higher, not lower, Parkinson's disease risk, and the association was more noticeable for lipophilic statins, an observation inconsistent with the current hypothesis that these statins protect nerve cells.'[12] How can the current view that statins protect nerve cells possibly have any possible currency, when nerve cells have the highest concentration of cholesterol of any cells in the body?

HOW STATINS CAUSE HARM

I have already mentioned that statins increased NO synthesis, which is a good thing. But the flip side is that they can also cause significant disruption to other key functions in the body. If this book has an underlying theme it is that everything in the human body is inter-connected.

You cannot simply pick off LDL with sniper fire, leaving everything else around it intact. When you fling a statin grenade into the body, you must expect that a whole bunch of different things will also take place – some good, some bad, some, so far, unknown. One of the major areas of collateral damage that was known by pharmaceutical companies, very early, is that statins not only block the manufacture of cholesterol, they also block the production of many other vital substances.

Cholesterol synthesis, as mentioned, is a 37-step process, but it is not a single road with a single end-point. The conversion of 3-hydroxy-3-methylglutaryl CoA into mevalonate happens very early on. It is step two.

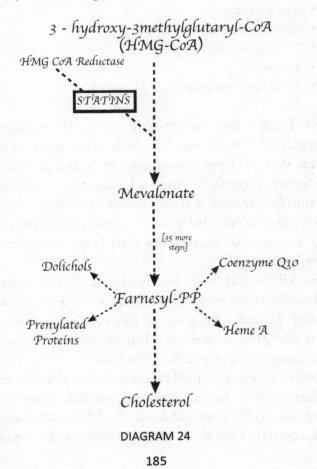

DIAGRAM 24

However, after this, mevalonate does not become cholesterol along one straight road. Mevalonate can then head off in many different directions, with many different destinations. When you block mevalonate production you also block the synthesis of many other critical substances. Here are some:

- Co-enzyme Q10
- Dolichols
- Tau proteins
- Seleno-proteins
- Nuclear Factor-Kappa B
- Heme A
- Prenylated proteins

Yes, I agree, they don't exactly trip off the tongue but I like to think of it this way. The body is not going to expend a great deal of energy synthesising these things unless they are highly important. After all, mammals switched off vitamin C synthesis and that is vital for life. Ergo, is it reasonable to expect that you can significantly deplete all the substances on that list, without there being some significant physiological cost?

You will be glad to know that I not going to discuss them all. Frankly, I have no idea what some of them do, e.g. seleno-proteins. Instead I am going to focus mainly on co-enzyme Q 10 (CoQ10), sometimes called ubiquinone because it *is* ubiquitous, found in all cells in the body.

CoQ10 is primarily used by the mitochondria, the energy-production units found in all cells, to make adenosine tri-phosphate (ATP). The breakdown of ATP to ADP (adenosine di-phosphate) is *the* single chemical process that powers all activity, in every cell in your body. Without it, nothing would happen and you'd immediately die.

It would be no exaggeration to say that synthesizing ATP is the most important chemical process in the body. It is the end-point of eating food, and you'd think anything that interferes with this activity is likely to have highly significant and damaging effects. Well that's the theory. What about reality? Do statins really interfere with CoQ10 synthesis?

Here is some research from Denmark. 'We have now shown that statin treatment affects the energy production in muscles. We are working on the assumption that this can be the direct cause of muscle weakness and pain in the patients. Scientists also showed that the patients examined who were being treated with statins had low levels of the key protein Q10. Q10 depletion and ensuing lower energy-production in the muscles could be the biological cause of the muscle pain that is a problem for many patients.'[13]

There is also a very rare genetic condition where people have low CoQ10 levels. When studied they were all found to have exercise intolerance, fatigue, muscle damage and pain, and high serum creatinine kinase.[14] Closer examination shows lipid accumulation and subtle signs of mitochondrial myopathy.

Creatinine kinase (CK) is an enzyme present in muscle cells. When the cells are damaged CK leaks out into the bloodstream, where it can be measured. If the levels get very high it means you are in danger of rhabdomyolysis. And statins significantly raise CK levels in many people because they damage muscles.

To quickly return to CoQ10. The most energy intense organ in your body is the heart, it beats away all day, every day, without rest. Could depletion of CoQ10, by blocking the production of ATP, lead to heart failure? Several researchers believe so. A couple of years ago a paper was written called 'Statins stimulate atherosclerosis and heart failure: pharmacological mechanisms' and stated that: 'In contrast to the current belief that cholesterol reduction with statins decreases atherosclerosis, we present a perspective that statins may be causative in coronary artery calcification and can function as mitochondrial toxins that impair muscle function in the heart and blood vessels through the depletion of coenzyme Q10 and 'heme A', and thereby ATP generation.'[15]

As the paper went on to say: 'With more than one million heart failure hospitalisations every year in the USA, the rapidly increasing prevalence of congestive heart failure is now described as an epidemic and is it likely that statin drug therapy is a major contributing factor.'

The pharmaceutical companies knew these things full well. Very early on, Merck filed a patent for a combination drug; a statin plus CoQ10 to be given simultaneously (US patent: 4,933,165.) They knew they had a problem with CoQ10, they had seen it in animal studies and pre-clinical trials. But in the end they chose not to pursue this.

Today we have been angrily informed that statins cause no side effects (more accurately called drug-related adverse effects) at all. Any adverse effects are due to the person taking the statin imagining they *will* get side effects, because they are told they might do so, the so-called nocebo effect. But ask yourself, does it not seem an amazing coincidence that the most common nocebo complaint of those taking statin is muscle pain and weakness. After all, we know that ...

- Statins dramatically lower CoQ10 levels
- People who have a rare genetic condition leading to low CoQ10 levels suffer from myopathy (muscle

weakness, pain and muscle cramps)
- Merck patented a CoQ10-statin combination (but did not use the patent)
- Statins are known to commonly raise an enzyme, which is also raised in muscle damage, called creatinine kinase (CK)
- Statins are known to cause rhabdomyolysis (severe breakdown of muscle cells)
- Patients taking statins often complain of muscle pain and weakness. Up to 60 per cent in some studies[16]

Knowing this, if you were going to expect one type of adverse effect from statins, muscle pain and weakness would be right at the top of the list. Yet muscle pain has been written off as a nocebo effect. Ladies and gentlemen of the jury, I put it to you that writing off patient-reported symptoms of muscle pain and weakness as the nocebo effect is medicine at its very, very worst. Paternalistic, dismissive, it flies in the face of the evidence.

And now for the dolichol pathway, and I'd estimate that approximately 0.001 per cent of doctors have heard of it. I certainly never had until I took a deeper interest in statins. If you want a more a technical discussion on what dolichols do, look on the spacedoc website.[17]

I am not going to dwell here for long because this is an enormously complex area, and requires knowledge of glycoproteins and vesicular shutting apparatus, and I cannot see any way of doing it in fewer than 50 pages. So I shall restrict this to saying that dolichols have critical functions in cell structure and cell signalling, and a low level of dolichols is associated with Parkinson's disease which, surprise, surprise, had recently been found to be associated with taking statins.[18]

In addition to the blocked pathways, we know that cholesterol itself is used to synthesise several further, downstream hormones. Vitamin D, oestrogen, cortisol, testosterone and the like. Again, the body doesn't make these for fun. Testosterone, for example. Here is one short section from the People's Pharmacy, a US website where people discuss adverse effects from drugs. 'Statins Sap Sex Drive and Lower Testosterone'. (Note: statins may have an overlooked side effect. Sexual dysfunction is not listed in the prescribing information, but many readers report low libido after taking statins.) 'I recently turned 50. I've been taking Livalo (pitavastatin) for high cholesterol and have been experiencing symptoms like no sexual desire. In addition, I can't sleep through the night, feel totally exhausted and have missed several days of work.'[19]

Statins lower cholesterol, cholesterol is required to synthesise testosterone, testosterone is critical for male sexual function. Why *wouldn't* statins reduce libido? It is exactly what you would expect them to do, once you understand their mode of action. Another nocebo effect, no doubt.

Personally, knowing exactly what they do, I cannot believe anyone could take a statin without suffering some significant adverse effects. Yes, some people do seem to manage well, but they must possess the physiology of an ox. On the other hand, if you probe about adverse effects, most people agree that since starting statins various things have gone awry. Adverse effects that are usually, sadly, angrily dismissed by their doctors. My e-mail bulges with such stories.

My comment to patients now is that: 'Statins add fifteen years to your life? No, they don't make you live fifteen years longer, they just make you feel fifteen years older.' And we laugh and laugh. They think I am joking, but I mean it.

CHAPTER 12

The Diet-Heart Meme

I t is impossible to talk about CVD without getting bogged down in the diet-heart hypothesis. Everyone has heard of it. In its simplest form – if you eat too much fat, or saturated fat, this will raise the cholesterol level in your blood and you will die of heart disease. There are variations on this theme, but the basic concept is always the same. A bad, fatty diet causes CVD.

I call this the Diet-Heart Meme. It is one of those things that everyone just knows to be true. A meme, by the way, is defined as 'An element of a culture or system of behaviour passed from one individual to another by imitation or other non-genetic means.' I think of a meme slightly differently, as an idea that has infiltrated the minds of everyone so thoroughly and completely it becomes almost impossible to shift. It didn't get there by a careful analysis of evidence, and evidence has no impact on it.

Medicine has had many terrible memes over the years. Ideas based on no evidence whatsoever, yet have become so widely believed that to question them is likely to result in banishment from the profession. I have tried to look for patterns in medical memes, and I think I have spotted a few:

- They should fit within existing belief systems
- They should be superficially simple and easy to understand
- They have a strong emotional appeal
- They appear to provide the answer to a pressing medical need

This fits with H. L. Mencken's observation that 'For every complex problem there is an answer that is clear, simple and wrong.'

The diet-heart hypothesis, in whatever form it now exists, is not new. It is getting on for 200 years old. However, not much attention was paid to it until the end of World War II when it seemed that suddenly, from nowhere, middle-aged men were keeling over and dying of heart attacks. This started in the US before spreading around much of the Western world.

Did heart attacks suddenly start after World War II? No. However, the rate of heart attacks was clearly at its peak in the US around that time. It triggered a widespread panic. What is causing this? What can we do?

Enter a man called Ancel Keys, one of those hugely energetic and charismatic figures who seems capable of convincing all those around him that he has *the* answer. He was helped at the time by the fact there was no real competing ideas, so he was pushing against an open door. However, I still marvel at the ability of some people to inspire and lead world opinion. Pity he inspired and led world opinion in the wrong direction. Oh well.

At the time, he knew one big thing – with no research data to back him up – that a diet high in cholesterol raised the cholesterol level in the blood and caused heart attacks. Sorry, rewind. He rapidly discovered that cholesterol in the diet has no impact on blood cholesterol levels.

After a short pause he found that he just knew something else, with similar conviction –that animal/saturated fats in the diet raised the cholesterol level and caused heart disease. With relentless energy he then went about proving it and, despite that fact that his research was horribly flawed, he succeeded. Or at least he succeeded to the satisfaction of a highly uncritical audience.

By 1961 Ancel Keys felt able to state: 'No other variable in the mode of life beside the fat calories in the diet is known which shows such constant relationship to the mortality rate from coronary or degenerative heart disease.' He later appeared on the cover of *Time* magazine as Mr Cholesterol. You, the man.

And that is pretty much where we remain today. Still stuck with the unchangeable meme that cannot be destroyed. 'That diet-heart hypothesis is out there! It can't be bargained with. It can't be reasoned with. It doesn't feel pity, or remorse or fear. And it absolutely will not stop ... ever, until you are dead!' (With apologies to Arnold Schwarzenegger.)

The advantage of the diet-heart hypothesis is that it ticks all the boxes in the clear and simple category. It is easy to visualise. We eat fat, we get fat, fat enters our bloodstream and gunks up our arteries. It also slots nicely into our existing prejudices. Most people don't like looking at fat, in any form. This creates a powerful emotional engagement with the hypothesis. On the other hand, look at a shiny apple or a crisp, steamed vegetable. They look healthy and by golly they must *be* healthy. How could anyone possibly believe that fat could be good for you, and fruit bad for you? What sort of a numpty is that?

Well, ahem, that'd be me.

The reality is that, if you spend some time studying the physiology of fatty acids, lipoproteins, etc., you quickly find that the entire diet-heart hypothesis starts to disintegrate in front of your very eyes. Having said this, due to the endless adaptations, it can be difficult to know what you are attacking. So, I shall reset the hypothesis. If you eat saturated fat this will cause your LDL level to rise – followed by CVD. Now, first question …

Why would eating substance A lead to an increase of substance B in the bloodstream? (If anything is unclear, go back to my explanations about the structure of saturated, polyunsaturated and monounsaturated fats, and what LDL is and where it comes from.) In other words, what possible reason could there be for the body to increase the concentration of LDL if you eat one type of fatty acid rather than another?

The current explanation is as follows. If you eat a lot of saturated fatty acids, and only saturated fatty acids, your body will reduce the number of LDL receptors causing the LDL level to rise (rather like mild FH). Whilst this is, superficially, a more sophisticated explanation than eating too much of A causes B to rise, it fails miserably to answer the question. What possible reason could there be for the body to 'downregulate' LDL receptor synthesis when confronted with a high consumption of saturated fatty acids?

I have never seen any cogent explanation for this. I have seen putative mechanisms of action, but no attempt to understand the underlying reason. It makes no sense from any physiological or biochemical perspective. Cholesterol and fats, saturated or otherwise, are not related to each other, except through the most indirect route. They sit together within LDL, and that is about that. But I do not wish to get drawn down too far into this sink-hole, for it goes around and around, and you never emerge. Time, instead, to focus on what happens to fatty acids after they are eaten.

First, they bind to cholesterol in the gut, are then absorbed through the gut wall, are packed together to make up triglycerides before the triglycerides are packed into chylomicrons. Then the chylomicrons head straight off into the bloodstream without, and this is important, passing through the liver. As mentioned before, they have their own private route into the bloodstream. The thoracic duct.

As chylomicrons pass through various organs, and float alongside cells, mainly fat cells, they are stripped of triglycerides and shrink down and down until the remaining chylomicron remnant is absorbed into the liver. There will be some fatty acids within the remnant that is taken up by the liver. But the clear majority of fat that you eat has nothing to do with the liver or LDL. It goes straight into fat cells to be stored. In times of energy need it will released from the fat cells as FFAs.

At this point, I need to remind everyone that the only source of LDL is VLDL. VLDLs, unlike chylomicrons, are made in the liver and then sent out in the blood. As with chylomicrons, they lose triglyceride as they pass fat cells, shrinking down to become LDLs. LDL is then removed from the bloodstream by LDL receptors on the liver, or other cells that need the cholesterol contained within LDL.

Where is the connection between the consumption of fatty acids and LDL, or LDL receptors? No, there is none.

This does, however, lead to the next question. Where do the fatty acids come from that make up the triglycerides, which are then packed into VLDLs? A small number will have arrived from the chylomicron remnants. Some will have arrived as FFAs that float about in the blood and get taken up by the liver. However, the majority of fatty acids are synthesised on site, in a process known as de novo lipogenesis (DNL).

The primary substance(s) used for DNL is clearly not fat, as fatty acids already are fats/lipids. No, the lipids manufactured in the liver come from the simple sugars, fructose and glucose. Whatever carbs you eat – pasta, bread, fruit, table sugar, vegetables, rice, cornflakes, etc. – they are all broken down into simple sugars in the gut.

After absorption these simple sugars travel straight from the gut to liver. When they reach the liver, one of four things can happen. First, they can be stored there as glycogen (lots of glucose molecules stuck together, end to end). Second, they can be released into the blood to be used for energy. Third, they can be taken up by muscle cells and stored there as local, muscle, glycogen stores. The average human can store about 1,500 calories of glycogen in total. Around 500 calories in the liver and 1,000 in muscles. Once these stores are full, if you keep on consuming carbs, beyond your immediate energy needs, the liver will now carry out the remaining, fourth function. It will convert the excess glucose and fructose into fatty acids.

Now, and here comes the most interesting part. The fatty acids synthesised in the liver are *saturated* fatty acids. This fact is worth repeating, then tattooing onto the forehead of every nutritionist alive. 'The liver synthesises saturated fatty acids.' They can be of different lengths but by far the most prevalent is palmitic acid, with a chain of 16 carbon atoms.

I mention this fact because palmitic acid is generally condemned as the most dangerous of all saturated fatty acids. *The* most likely to cause CVD. Why, because it has been found in higher tissue concentrations in people with a greater risk of CVD. This, of course, represents an almost perfect irony.

We find higher concentrations of palmitic acid in people at higher risk of CVD, then state that we should restrict the consumption of palmitic acid. However, the palmitic acid we find will almost certainly have come from excess carbohydrate consumption. Ergo, it is a high carbohydrate consumption that is damaging, *not* a high palmitic acid consumption. If this wasn't all so stupid and damaging, it would be funny.

Of equal, perhaps even greater, importance is the fact that of the two simple sugars, the one that is preferentially turned into saturated fat is fructose. In fact, it seems that no fructose is released from the liver into the bloodstream. Which, in turn, means you cannot have a blood fructose level. What we measure in the blood, in diabetes and suchlike, is only the blood glucose level. Potentially, therefore, it is fructose we should be most concerned about. After consumption and digestion, it travels straight to the liver where it is converted to fatty acid/palmitic acid. Do not pass the liver, do not collect £200.

It has been proposed that, over time, overconsumption of fructose will lead to a condition known as non-alcoholic fatty liver disease (NAFLD) as the liver starts to engorge with too much fat. NAFLD can lead on to cirrhosis, liver failure and death. This condition is now becoming a virtual epidemic in

West. Where do we get fructose from? The answer is sucrose/table sugar, most soft drinks, high fructose corn syrup and, of course, fruit.

Whilst it is difficult, if not impossible to see how eating fat – of any type – will affect VLDL synthesis, and thus LDL levels. It is basic human physiology, page one, paragraph one, to work out how eating excess carbs will raise VLDL levels and, ironically, saturated fatty acid levels around the body.

Nor, I hasten to add, do I believe that the high concentration of fatty acids in cells around the body cause any problem. I refuse to believe that the liver is going to preferentially synthesise saturated fatty acids, if they are harmful to our health. Just in case you think this is all highly theoretical, this is exactly what does happen. After a high carb meal, de novo lipogenesis can easily rise seven times as high as after a high fat meal.[1] Then, in turn, the VLDL/triglyceride level rises far, far, higher.[2]

What you see is exactly what you would expect to see, once you understand how the human metabolic system works. It is all quite straightforward. It may explain why the American sugar industry has always been rather keen to spend money to manipulate research in this area.

An investigation a couple of years ago found that, in the 1960s, the American sugar industry paid Harvard researchers to produce a clinical paper stating that the cause of CVD was saturated fat intake, not sugar. In the UK this behaviour was eventually unearthed, and was reported in the *Daily Telegraph*: 'In 1964, the Sugar Association ... approved "Project 226", which entailed paying Harvard researchers today's equivalent of $48,900 for an article reviewing the scientific literature, supplying materials they wanted reviewed, and receiving drafts of the article.

'The resulting article ... concluded there was "no doubt" that reducing cholesterol and saturated fat was the only dietary intervention needed to prevent heart disease ...

'"Let me assure you this is quite what we had in mind and we look forward to its appearance in print," wrote an employee of the sugar industry to one of the authors.'[3]

Nowadays, I find it hard to believe a single bloody word that is written about heart disease and diet. In the 1970s, the UK researcher Professor John Yudkin realised that if we were looking for a dietary culprit in CVD, we should look at sugar not fat. His book was called *Pure, White and Deadly*. He was attacked and vilified from all sides, especially by Ancel Keys.

Here is another section from an article entitled 'The sugar conspiracy'.

> Robert Lustig is a paediatric endocrinologist at the University of California who specialises in the treatment of childhood obesity. A 90-minute talk he gave in 2009, titled 'Sugar: The Bitter Truth', has now been viewed more than six million times on YouTube. In it, Lustig argues forcefully that fructose, a form of sugar ubiquitous in modern diets, is a 'poison' culpable for America's obesity epidemic.
>
> A year or so before the video was posted, Lustig gave a similar talk to a conference of biochemists in Adelaide, Australia. Afterwards, a scientist in the audience approached him. Surely, the man said, you've read Yudkin. Lustig shook his head. John Yudkin, said the scientist, was a British professor of nutrition who had sounded the alarm on sugar back in 1972, in a book called *Pure, White, and Deadly*.

'If only a small fraction of what we know about the effects of sugar were to be revealed in relation to any other material used as a food additive,' wrote Yudkin, 'that material would promptly be banned.' The book did well, but Yudkin paid a high price for it. Prominent nutritionists combined with the food industry to destroy his reputation, and his career never recovered. He died, in 1995, a disappointed, largely forgotten man.[4]

You don't need to be a green-ink-writing-conspiracy theorist to believe that there is a worldwide conspiracy to attack and silence anyone who dares to suggest that sugar, and especially fructose, may not be the healthiest substance around. Those who take on the sugar industry and soft-drink manufacturers are still being destroyed. Perhaps the most well known is Professor Tim Noakes.

'An American may not be able to grasp what Tim Noakes means to South Africa since no equivalent to Professor Noakes exists in the US. In South Africa, Noakes is a nationally famous exercise scientist and physician who has transformed the practice of sport by challenging most commonly held beliefs. And yet, Noakes' own university and colleagues, along with the medical establishment, have suddenly turned against him in what he describes as his "final crusade." Having demolished dogma on subjects as diverse as hydration, motivation and fatigue, Noakes may have gone a step too far. *He took on carbs.*'[5]

For suggesting that a high-carb diet may be the primary cause of obesity and diabetes he has been dragged to court once, where South Africa's council for health professionals met to decide whether he should keep his medical licence. Noakes won, but at the time of writing he is going to be dragged to court again.

Win or lose, other researchers will look at what happened and is happening to Tim Noakes, and wonder if it is worth criticising sugar. The answer is almost certainly no. Having said this, I am certainly not as ferociously anti-carb as some. In fact, I started life at the other end of the spectrum. I was looking for evidence that animal fatty acids/saturated fatty acids caused CVD. I could find none. Or, at least, I could not find any that was not of extremely poor quality. In time I began to recognise that, if we were looking for a dietary culprit, excess carbs were sitting there with an evil grin.

I would add that not everyone has a problem with carbs, and I am not suggesting that fruit and vegetables are unhealthy and should be avoided at all costs. Frankly, that would be ridiculous. However, if your diet is based on crisps, bread, pasta, sugary soft drinks and you glug down half a pint of fruit juice whilst liberally sprinkling sugar on your breakfast cereal, then do not expect that eating an apple is going to keep you healthy. It is going to make things worse. And do not rely on diet soft drinks to keep you thin.

The reality is that there is a point, and I do not know where that point is, because it is different for everyone, where carbs can become a major problem, and fructose is a very specific problem if taken in quantity. On the other hand, fat and saturated fat are perfectly healthy. I could include study after study demonstrating this but will stick to just one because it was massive, very recent and was set up by Professor Salim Yusuf, who can in no way be considered a maverick researcher. Look him up.

The trial in question was the Prospective Urban Rural

Epidemiology study (PURE). It involved eighteen countries and 135,000 people, studied over seven years.

PURE STUDY, DIRECTLY CONTRADICTORY TO RECENT AHA ADVISORY

'The saturated-fat findings will be particularly controversial, especially in the cardiology community, which has traditionally held the mantra that saturated fat is the number one dietary enemy.

'Indeed, just a few weeks ago, the American Heart Association issued a new "advisory" recommending minimizing intake of saturated fat and replacing it with polyunsaturated fat or carbohydrate. The PURE findings appear to be in direct contradiction to this advice.

'Commenting on this at her hotline presentation, PURE co-lead author Dr Mahshid Dehghan (McMaster University) said: "The upper levels of saturated fat intake in our study (mean 10%–13% of dietary energy) was associated with a significantly reduced mortality compared with low levels of saturated fat, and *very low saturated-fat intake appears harmful.* Current guidelines that recommend total fat below 30% and saturated fat below 10% of energy intake are not supported by our data."

'Yusuf commented further: "*The AHA guidelines are not based on the best evidence* – saturated fat was labelled as a villain years ago, and the traditional church has kept on preaching that message. They have been resistant to change."'

The final comment on PURE stated that: 'PURE study's findings broadly support the notion that reducing total fat intake may be unwarranted and that *replacing saturated fat intake with (refined) carbohydrates is not a good recipe for cardiovascular health.*'[6]

It's also worth mentioning that a couple of years ago I was greatly amused by the fact that Credit Suisse, not an organisation you would necessarily turn to for nutritional advice, carried out a massive research project on diet and health. This was done to advise investors about new trends in food production and where to invest their money.

With regard to saturated fat, they concluded that: 'Based on medical and our own research we can conclude that the intake of saturated fat (butter, palm and coconut oil and lard) poses no risk to our health and particularly to the heart. In the words of probably the most important epidemiological study published on the subject by Siri-Tarino et al: "There is no significant evidence for concluding that dietary saturated fat is associated with an increased risk of CHD or CVD." Saturated fat is actually a healthy source of energy.'[7]

Of course, their report was inevitably rubbished and dismissed. What do bankers know about cardiology? Who are these idiots? Well, they weren't all bankers. Most of those involved in this report were medics, or medical researchers, working for them. And whilst I hold no candle for investment bankers, I do know that they are the least sentimental people on the planet. They simply do facts, evidence and money, and they can strip an argument down to bare bones faster than a shoal of piranha.

The obesity and diabetes epidemic

There is, of course, another argument commonly used against fat consumption, not directly related to CVD. For many years, it has been stated that eating fat makes you fat. The main basis for this claim is that fat contains twice as many calories per gram as carbohydrates. If you eat 100g of fat this will provide you with 900 kilocalories of energy, whereas 100g of carbohydrate will give you around 450 kilocalories.

It is inarguable that, if you eat the same number of grams of carbohydrate as fat, you will consume fewer calories and are less likely to become obese. However, most people do not eat grams of food. They eat pretty much what they like, and do not exchange one type of food for another, unless, that is, they attend the likes of Weight Watchers. And then there is the linked argument against fat, which is that eating fat not only makes you obese, but becoming obese causes diabetes and diabetes greatly increases the risk of CVD. If you believe that saturated fat has its own, unique CVD-causing properties, you will be even more concerned about people with diabetes eating fat. Therefore, the current advice for those with diabetes is to eat a high-carb, low-fat (HCLF) diet.

And from such simple, some may say simplistic thinking, the healthy eating guidelines emerged in the US and UK. These guidelines have a nasty habit of flipping about in front of your eyes, but their ineluctable essence remains much the same. Eat less fat, especially saturated fat, and consume more healthy carbs, e.g. pasta, rice, bread, etc. You may have seen various versions of the eat-well plate, or the food pyramid. This is the original 1992 version.

DIAGRAM 25

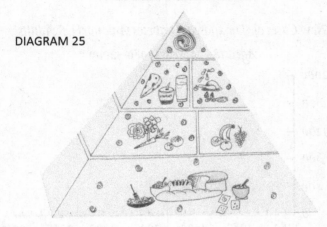

There is only one slight problem with this. Since the introduction of the healthy eating guidelines, the eat-well plate and food pyramid, the rates of obesity and diabetes have not fallen. In fact, there has been an inexorable rise in both.

Overweight and Obesity

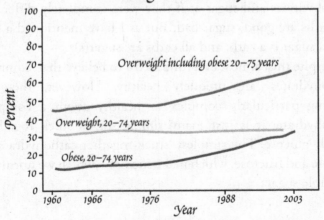

SOURCES: Centers for Disease Control and Prevention, National Center for Health Statistics, Health, United States, 2006, Figure 13.

DIAGRAM 26

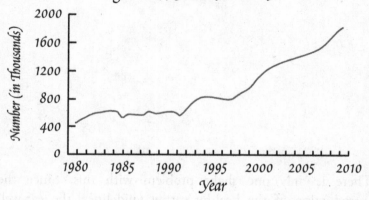

New Cases of Diagnosed Diabetes Among U.S Adults Aged 18–79 Years 1980–2009

SOURCE: http://www.cdc.gov/diabetes/statistics/incidence/fig1.htm.

DIAGRAM 27

Just to provide a little additional context, everyone talks about carbohydrates and sugar as if they were completely different, i.e. carbs are good, sugar bad. But as I have mentioned a few times, sugar is a carb, and all carbs are sugar(s).

Despite this, almost everyone seems to believe that 'complex carbohydrates' are uniquely healthy. However, there is nothing particularly complex or healthy about a complex carbohydrate; it is just many simple sugars stuck together, mainly glucose. The simplest 'stuck-together carbohydrate' is glucose and fructose, which make sucrose – which we normally call table sugar.

Glucose

Fructose

Sucrose

If you continue to link simple sugars together you end up with more and more complex carbs, such as chitin and cellulose, which make up as the likes of lobster shells and trees. Yes, a tree is, in large part, millions of sugar molecules chemically bound together. A wooden ski chalet is a big sugar cube. However, wood, grass and most vegetables have their sugars bound together so strongly that the bonds are difficult to break down, and our puny human digestive systems cannot deal with them at all.

If we eat wood, it passes straight through. In fact, if we eat most vegetables they pass straight through and out the other end. Yes, healthy fibre. On that basis you might as well eat a brick. Most of the grains and vegetables that we eat must be heated for a considerable length of time to break down most of the bonds, before our digestive systems can do the final work. Try eating a raw potato, a raw kidney bean or uncooked wheat to see how well we digest most vegetables and grain. You can sit on the toilet and view the scene if you like. Indeed, you probably *will* have to sit on the toilet.

The main point I want to emphasise is that every carb you consume will, if your gut can manage it, be turned into a simple sugar, before absorption. So, if you eat bread, you are eating sugar. If you eat pasta, the same. Ditto rice and fruit. If you eat vegetables you are, primarily, eating sugar.

If you look at the food pyramid or the healthy-eating plate in this light, you can see that it is essentially a pyramid or a plate of sugar. Call it a pyramid of carbs if that makes you feel better. Yes, there are minerals and vitamins and proteins and some vegetable fats in there too, which are necessary for life. But it is still, primarily, sugar.

Having said this, you could spend your entire life consuming nothing but the items on the healthy-eating plate and remain fit and healthy, and live to 100. However, many people do not do well on the eat-well plate, which is something that Professor Tim Noakes found out for himself. He was a long-distance runner who followed the healthy-eating guidelines, yet still he became overweight and diabetic. Which rather pissed him off.

He was doing everything he had been told was good for him. He was moving more, eating less, eating healthily and it DID NOT WORK. Ironically, he was doing everything he had advised other people to do, as he was a well-respected nutritional scientist.

He wanted to know why, so he studied the area with fresh eyes. He looked at the evidence from a difference angle and concluded that the carbohydrates were causing the problem. So, he put himself on a high-fat, low carb (HFLC) diet. He lost weight and his diabetes reversed, then disappeared. When he felt that he needed to pass this message on to the world he then got the full Yudkin treatment.

What Tim Noakes' story highlights is that, for a significant number of people, the main reason why they get fat and develop diabetes is because they are eating too much sugar ... sorry, carbs. The irony is that this is exactly what they were told to do to remain thin and healthy. Oh well.

This whole sad situation is made far worse in those who go on to develop type 2 diabetes. In diabetes, one of the main problems, perhaps the central problem, is an inability to control blood sugar levels. This is despite producing enough insulin, sometimes a very high level of insulin, which is why the underlying disease process is often called insulin resistance. (A term that I shall let pass without further comment here.)

Logic dictates that if you have insulin resistance and very high blood sugar levels, the best advice must be to eat fewer carbs. Instead, people with diabetes are given the exact opposite message. They are told to avoid fat and eat carbs.

I would only disagree with that statement in the following ways:

- Eating fat does not make you fat
- Eating fat does not cause diabetes
- Eating carbs makes you fat
- Eating carbs causes diabetes
- Eating fat does not increase the risk of CVD
- Eating carbs increases the risk of CVD

Apart from that, everything else is tickety-boo. But despite the inescapable, metabolic logic, the HFLC v LFHC war continues to rage. On the low-fat side are the key opinion leaders, the diabetes societies, the food and pharmaceutical industries, the guideline writers and the vegans. On the other side sit ... everyone who is capable of understanding science.

Debating with the anti-fat, pro-carb brigade can become somewhat tedious. To quote Mark Twain, 'Never argue with stupid people, they will drag you down to their level and then beat you with experience.'

And now to return to Credit Suisse, this time looking at the risk of diabetes and obesity in the last thirty years or so. 'Saturated fat has not been a driver of obesity: fat does not make you fat. At current levels of consumption, the most likely culprit behind growing obesity level of the world population is *carbohydrates* ... please note that *carbohydrates and vegetable oils accounted for over 90% of the increase in calorie intake in this period.*

Healthcare officials and government bodies have been consistently behind developments on the research front ... We would also expect a review at some point of the neutral stance on carbohydrates; *carbohydrates are one if not the major cause behind the fast growth of metabolic syndrome cases in the US – 4% a year – which includes type 2 diabetes and obesity.'*

You could ask why I'm quoting Credit Suisse on scientific matters again. Well, to repeat, they came to health and nutrition with no dog in the race. They are also fully capable of understanding science, because that is what they do. And their findings carry no bias, which is more can than can be said for those who bellow at each other from either side of the fat/carbohydrate swamp.

Of course, you can find hundreds of articles in peer-reviewed nutrition journals, 'proving' that carbs, especially fructose, have nothing to do with obesity and diabetes. For example, here is a paper entitled 'Controversies about sugars: results from systematic reviews and meta-analyses on obesity, cardiometabolic disease and diabetes', published in the *European Journal of Nutrition*.[8]

The main conclusion was that: 'Despite the continuing concern regarding fructose's unique metabolic effects, which stems from low-quality ecological studies, animal models and select human studies, the highest level of evidence from systematic review and meta-analysis does not support a direct causal relationship with cardiometabolic disease.'

In short, fructose is fine, no problem, move along. But is it possible that the authors have some conflict of interest? In fact, the conflict of interest statement at the end of this article is far too long to reproduce in full. However, disclosed conflicts of interest include:

- Tate and Lyle
- Dr Pepper Snapple group
- The Coca-Cola company
- The European Fruit Juice Association

You can also find this statement: 'This article belongs to a supplement sponsored by Rippe Health.' Who, I wondered, are Rippe Health? Well ... 'Rippe Health Evaluation and Rippe Lifestyle Institute are the world leaders in Lifestyle Medicine research including nutrition, weight management and physical activity as well as heart disease prevention, publishing and multimedia.'[9] And who are their sponsors? They include:

- Kraft
- Coca-Cola
- Welch's

- Dr Pepper Snapple
- AstraZeneca
- General Mills
- 100% Pure Florida (fruit juice)
- Corn Refiners' association
- McDonald's
- Kellogg's
- Lilly
- Pfizer
- Roche
- Johnson and Johnson [etc.]

Now, I still don't really know who Rippe Health are, but I most certainly do now know who their sponsors are. As for no evidence about fructose: here is a graph, looking at de novo lipogenesis (DNL) in the liver following a glucose 'meal' v a fructose 'meal'.[10]

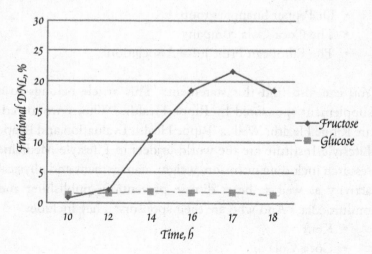

DIAGRAM 29

If you are a scientist, a graph like that tells you absolutely everything you need to know about the impact of fructose v glucose on the human body. The effect of fructose on fat creation/storage is probably why many hibernating animals stock up on as much fruit as they can, before falling asleep for six months. The fructose in fruit makes them fat, and being fat allows them to survive six months fast asleep. Ain't nature wonderful.

I shall end this section by looking at two medical doctors and their experiences with the HFLC diet. The first is a friend and colleague who had a damascene conversion, similar to Tim Noakes, a few years ago. He hated, absolutely hated, dealing with obese and overweight patients in his practice. He told them all to exercise more, eat less and avoid fats. But his success rate using the advice was zero.

He referred patients to dieticians, hoping they would then leave him alone. But as night follows day, they would all come back, even more obese, with even higher blood sugar levels. At which point he started them on various medications to keep their blood sugar under control. With wearisome inevitability they simply got fatter and fatter, and their blood sugars rose even higher.

In the final throw of the polypharmacy diabetic dice, he added insulin to their drug regime – and watched things get even worse. He could do nothing for them. He found it terribly stressful and dispiriting. He scrutinised the value of his NHS pension on-line and was planning his retirement, so fed up had he become.

Then one day a lady arrived at his surgery for an appointment. She has been obese, now was slim. He asked her what she had done. At first she was reluctant to tell him as she thought he would strongly disapprove. Now, Dr David Unwin is the least disapproving man you could ever meet. He is the perfect, amiable vicar who loves his flock with unwavering humanity. He makes me look like Donald Trump. He will curl up with embarrassment when he reads this.

Eventually the patient revealed to him that, as a last resort, she had tried a HFLC diet. For the first time in her life she lost weight, and the weight had stayed off. David was sorely tempted to dismiss her as a fruitcake. But he was intrigued. He went home, he started reading, researching; he even read my book.

He then tried the HFLC diet himself. He found that he had fewer hunger cravings and more energy. Although he had never been fat, or even overweight, he lost a few pounds in weight. So he tried the diet with some of his intractably obese patients, and almost immediately achieved amazing results. Blood sugar levels fell, weight dropped off – and stayed off. He roped in some other members of staff, and they too saw immediate benefits.

Today, he has a fully low-carb practice. His partners, who were initially sceptical, have bought into the idea. He began to record the data on his patients, demonstrating both long-term weight loss and diabetic control. Many of his diabetic patients have even been 'cured', in so much as their blood sugar levels are now well within the normal range.

His practice now spends less on diabetic medications than any surrounding practice, and their prescribing costs for diabetes are going down, whilst everywhere else in the country the amount they spend is going through the roof. Read his journey of discovery in the *Diabetes Times*.[11] His research, showing weight loss over the longer term, control of diabetes and greatly improved liver function has been published for all to see.[12]

Yet, despite his work and the work of any high-fat low-carbers, it remains a medical heresy to promote an HFLC diet. The establishment is still ready and willing to release the dementors, to terrorise anyone who suggests it may be beneficial.

Meanwhile, in Australia, the orthopaedic surgeon Gary Fettke was silenced by the Australian Health Practitioners Regulatory Authority (AHPRA) for daring to advise patients to eat fewer carbs and more fat. He had been struggling to operate on obese patients, and wondered if anything could be done to help them lose weight. He too found that the HFLC diet worked. His tale is both hilarious and deeply upsetting. His wife is now blogging on his behalf.[13]

Following various hearings Gary Fettke was warned that, even if his views become accepted medical practice, he will not be allowed to talk about them to any patient – ever. Which is perhaps the most stupid judgement in the history of medical authority, and that takes some doing. A doctor unable to tell his patients about best medical practice.

> Patient: 'Tell me, Dr Fettke, what do you think I should eat to help me lose weight and control my diabetes?
>
> Dr Fettke: 'I am sorry I am not allowed to talk to you about such matters, for I am a mere orthopaedic surgeon who cannot understand such complex things. For that you must talk to a dietician.'

Yes, really.

Having said this, I must reiterate that vegetarians can be perfectly healthy. Vegans can also be perfectly healthy – so long as they take the required vitamin supplements. Carbs are not unhealthy per se. Your body can use sugar for energy, it can store excess sugar as fat and then use that for energy. A lot of people seem perfectly able to deal with a high-carb diet.

However, many people struggle badly with too many carbs. They put on weight, develop fatty livers and become insulin resistant. They can develop full-blown non-alcoholic fatty liver disease (NAFLD), which can, in extreme cases, lead to liver failure. These things will improve, in some cases disappear, if they switch to a HFLC diet.

Therefore, the general healthy advice on nutrition is ...

If in doubt – eat fat.

CHAPTER 13

Does Raised Cholesterol (LDL) Cause CVD?

I toyed with the idea of making this the shortest chapter in the book. In one short word ... NO! Which needs a quick explanation.

Whilst more and more people seem perfectly content to accept that a high-fat/saturated-fat (or high-cholesterol) diet is not a cause of CVD, almost everyone remains stuck firmly with the high blood cholesterol meme. I am always tempted to ask them how can a hypothesis survive when its legs have been chopped off?

Leaving that issue aside. I realise it is difficult to accept that something so widely believed and supported by all the experts, guidelines writers, government agencies, doctors, researchers and anyone else you can think of can be wrong. But it is. It began as one of these horribly seductive ideas that starts with no scientific basis, but then gathers scientific justification around itself in endless post-hoc rationalisation. When flatly contradicted, it simply reforms and carries on.

As stated several times now, but it bears repeating, the overall cholesterol hypothesis started out very simply. If you eat too much cholesterol, the cholesterol level in your blood will rise and that excess cholesterol will be deposited into your artery walls, causing atherosclerotic plaques to form.

The first problem to emerge, as noted by Ancel Keys, is that cholesterol in the diet has little or no impact on the cholesterol level in your bloodstream. Undeterred, Keys simply adjusted the hypothesis. It became fat *and* cholesterol. In most cases, if you are eating animal produce, you will be eating both fat and cholesterol, so the data can never be disentangled, which is a good way to protect a poorly formed hypothesis from direct attack, but very poor science.

Recently, the US dietary guidelines advisory committee proposed that dietary cholesterol should be removed as a 'nutrient of concern'. In other words, dietary cholesterol has nothing to do with CVD. They managed to work this out a mere seventy years after Keys first noticed any association between dietary and blood cholesterol.

Unsurprisingly, the US Dietary Committee was attacked for daring to make this statement, mainly by the Physicians Committee for Responsible Medicine in 'The Physicians Committee sues USDA and DHHS, Exposing Industry Corruption in Dietary Guidelines Decision on Cholesterol.'[1]

It is to be noted that the committee's website lists their priorities, which include shifting research from animal 'models' to human-relevant studies and working with policy-makers and industry to adopt alternatives to chemical tests on animals.

Although the dietary part of the cholesterol hypothesis has pretty much disappeared, the cholesterol part continues unaffected. Or does it? In fact, it has also constantly swirled and adapted, and altered many times.

When Keys, and others, first came up with the high blood cholesterol hypothesis no one knew that cholesterol was carried about in lipoproteins of different sizes and shapes. Your cholesterol level was simply an amalgamation of many different lipoproteins jumbled together – VLDL, IDL, LDL and HDL.

It was not until 1950 that LDL was discovered.[2] At which point LDL became *the* lipoprotein to be worried about. Which means that Ancel Keys knew that high cholesterol levels caused CVD when he didn't even know there were different types of lipoprotein, and only one of them, LDL, is thought to be damaging. In short, he didn't even know what a *high* cholesterol level was.

But you cannot let a little thing like completely failing to understand how cholesterol is carried in the blood damage your hypotheses. It simply meant another change. Fat/saturated fat, plus or minus cholesterol, raises the LDL level (not the total cholesterol level) in your bloodstream. This then causes atherosclerotic plaques to form.

However, this hypothesis has since undergone many further adaptations. Some LDL is now considered 'good' because it is light and fluffy, whereas small and dense LDL is 'bad'. Many doctors have even moved onto measuring the LDL particle number LDLp rather that LDLc (LDL-cholesterol). Others have become more interested in the Apo A to Apo B ratio, or oxidised rather than non-oxidised LDL. There is also the concept of dyslipidaemia, including VLDL and HDL ratio. I could go on. This hypothesis constantly swirls and mutates before your eyes.

As any scientist knows, if your hypothesis needs to constantly adapt to fit the facts, it is a completely rubbish hypothesis. Or, put another way, it is not actually a hypothesis but a reactive collation of facts. Endless adaptations cannot transform it into a predictive model. It just becomes an ever more confusing mess.

Despite this flurry of Brownian motion, one point just about manages to stand firm amidst the chaos, which is the belief that LDL causes CVD, small and dense, oxidised or not. This belief rests on three pillars of evidence.

- People with raised LDL levels are more likely to die of CVD
- If you lower LDL levels with statins the risk of CVD is reduced
- Those with FH are far more likely to die of CVD, and at a young age

Unfortunately, at this point I am going to switch back and forward between talking about the total cholesterol and LDL. The reason for this is that, in many countries, and over time, the LDL level has not been measured separately from the total cholesterol level. This means that for various populations, it is only the total cholesterol level that I have figures for. However, the total cholesterol level acts as a pretty good proxy for LDL. Normally, if the total cholesterol is 5mmol/l, the LDL will be close to 3mmol/l. (This ratio falls apart in FH.)

The first question that needs to be answered is, what is a raised cholesterol or LDL level? You may think this is a strange one to ask. Surely, we must now by know what it is? Well, we do not. I can tell you the average cholesterol level in the UK, the US or France. They are similar, but not the same. As for telling you what is a high cholesterol level, that's tricky.

For example, a high cholesterol level in the UK is currently considered to be anything over 5mmol/l. In the US it is 200mg/dl – they use alternative units in the US – and 200mg/dl equates to 5.2mmol/l. Why the difference between 5mmol/l and 5.2mmol/l? The only explanation I can find is that doctors like nice simple figures. 5mmol/l in Europe, 200mg/dl in the US.

Does this 0.2 difference matter? Well, I would imagine that there must be around ten million people in the US who have a cholesterol level between 5 and 5.2mmol/l, which means that there's one hell of a lot of people in the US with a cholesterol level normal for them that would be considered high, and in need of treatment, in Europe. Science at its finest.

However, that minor problem is swamped by the conundrum that at least 70 per cent of people, in most countries, have a cholesterol level above 5mmol/l. This means that the average level is not considered normal, it is high. Yes, logic warps and bends again, and there is another sinister crack in the structure of the universe.

Next question, who decided that 5mmol/l was high? This was decreed in 1984 at the US National Cholesterol Consensus Conference. There was no evidence then to support this completely arbitrary figure, and still isn't. It just is. I know you may find this difficult to believe, but it is true. To add to the confusion, if you have had a heart attack or stroke, anything above 4mmol/l is considered high and should be lowered. The same if you have diabetes. So, there are different levels for high – and needing treatment – for different people. In truth, the 'normal' cholesterol level is an ever-moving target that can never be pinned down.

Here, from the Harvard Medical School, is an article entitled 'LDL cholesterol: Low, lower, and lower still'.

The overall message on 'bad' LDL cholesterol is much the same as it has been: Lower is better and how low your level should be depends on your cardiovascular risk factors.

But the standard for what low LDL means keeps on getting lower. While an LDL level under 70 (1.8mmol/l) is still the usual goal for people at the highest risk for cardiovascular disease perhaps that is still too high.

Over the past 20 years as new evidence about LDL rolls in, experts have been pushing their recommendations about the 'ideal' LDL level lower and lower.

We're not there yet, but perhaps someday there will be a consensus that nearly everyone should make aggressive attempts to lower their LDL cholesterol with statins. If the overall LDL recommendation were to become 50–70, taking a statin may become part of the daily health routine.[3]

If you follow their logic, that would mean aiming for a total cholesterol level of about 2.8 to 3.5mmol/l, lower than any human population ever discovered in the history of the world. Which means that every single person alive has a 'high' cholesterol level. In turn, this means that there can be no such thing as normal.

Low, lower and lower still. The general thinking now appears to have crystallised around the belief that LDL is like smoking. There is no safe amount, and zero would be the ultimate aim. Some have already set a new arbitrary target at 1mmol/l. Just like ... well, like those with Smith-Lemli-Opitz syndrome, the genetically inherited dysfunction of cholesterol synthesis. 'Smith-Lemli-Opitz syndrome is a developmental disorder characterised by distinctive facial features, small head size (microcephaly), intellectual disability or learning problems, and behavioral problems. Malformations of the heart, lungs, kidneys, gastrointestinal tract, and genitalia may also occur.'[4]

Without sufficient cholesterol, the foetus cannot develop properly and ends up horribly malformed, and are we really aiming to get everyone's LDL down to that level? Anyway, in answer to the initial question, what is a raised cholesterol or LDL level? The current, mainstream answer would seem to be – anything above zero. Whatever the level is, lower it further.

How does this fit with the evidence? Not very well, I would suggest. Let's start by having a look at Japan, the early poster boy for the diet-heart cholesterol hypothesis. When Ancel Keys was looking at countries around the world, Japan stood out as having the lowest fat intake, the lowest cholesterol levels and the lowest rate of heart disease. Bingo!

People have become a bit less vocal about Japan recently. Why would this be, I wonder? Primarily because over the last 50 years the average cholesterol level in Japan has risen and risen. At one time it was 3.9mmol/l. It is now 5.2mmol/l, which is about the same as the US, a bit lower than the UK and the same as, to pick another country at random, Canada.

As the average cholesterol level in Japan has risen steadily, the rate of death from heart disease has not followed suit. Instead it has fallen by 60 per cent. At the same time the rate of stroke has fallen seven-fold. Japan used to have just about the highest rate of strokes in the world, but it is now among the lowest. So, a 25 per cent rise in cholesterol levels has been accompanied by a six-fold drop in death from CVD.[5] I should add that fat consumption has also risen by 400 per cent in that period. Thus, we don't really talk about Japan so much any more.

There are those whose immediate solution to this contradictory evidence is to suggest that the Japanese are genetically protected from CVD, in some way, and therefore do not represent a paradox. No, they are not. Japanese emigrants to the US have the same level of CVD as the surrounding population.[6]

Maybe I should just leave things here. Explain Japan? Over 100 million direct and absolute contradictions to the cholesterol hypothesis. Not a black swan, a flying squadron of black elephants. They fly happily alongside the French Paradox. The French have the highest saturated-fat consumption in Europe, slightly higher than average cholesterol levels, and the lowest CVD rate in Europe. Nearly as low as Japan.

The simple fact is that there is absoutely no relationship between cholesterol levels in various countries and the rate of death from CVD. In the *Great Cholesterol Con* I used figures from the WHO MONICA study, some of which are worth repeating here.

- In 2009 the average cholesterol level for men, in France, was 5.9mmol/l. In Russia, which had the highest rate of CHD in Europe, it was 5.1mmol/l.
- Rates of death from coronary heart disease (CHD) per 100,000 a year in Russia and France were ...
  Russia = 267
  (cholesterol level 5.1mmol/l)
  France = 24 (cholesterol level 5.9mmol/l)

And just to bring in the country with the highest average cholesterol level:

- Switzerland = 32 (cholesterol level 6.4mmol/l)

Yes indeed, in 2009 the Swiss had the highest average cholesterol level of any country in the world, and the second lowest rate of death from CHD in Europe, about the fourth lowest in the world. Did they not know they should be dropping dead? Maybe sleeping next to tax-free gold bullion is good for you.

When you look at facts like this, the idea that cholesterol has anything to do with CVD seems the most complete nonsense. However, I know that people can, and will, say that you cannot compare different countries because there are many other confounding variables like blood pressure, rates of smoking, etc. Yes, I know all the arguments, I have heard them so many times I could recite them in my sleep. In fact, worryingly, I do.

However, researchers have also looked at cholesterol levels within counties and compared them with deaths from CVD. Some years ago, the investigators of a study in Norway contacted me to tell me about the results of their study. They analysed blood cholesterol levels in over 50,000 people over a fifteen-year period, in the HUNT2 study. Gratifyingly, they knew I was a bit of a cholesterol sceptic and wished to share their data with me. Fame at last. Yes, this study has been published, but such was the resounding worldwide silence you would never have known it.

They divided people into four groups. First, those with a cholesterol level of less than 5.0mmol/l, who they used as the reference point. They set the risk of ischaemic heart disease (IHD) mortality for this group at one. They then looked at the risk of dying of an MI in those with higher cholesterol levels, both men and women. When you look at the graph, the axis on the left is the hazard ratio (HR) (with apologies to all statisticians out there). An HR of 1.20 means a 20 per cent increased risk of death. An HR of 0.80 means a 20 per cent reduced risk of death, over the fifteen years of the study.

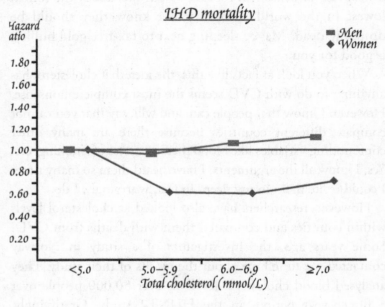

IHD mortality

■ Men
♦ Women

Hazard ratio

1.80
1.60
1.40
1.20
1.00
0.80
0.60
0.40
0.20

<5.0   5.0–5.9   6.0–6.9   ≥7.0
Total cholesterol (mmol/L)

DIAGRAM 30

As you can see, with men, as the cholesterol level rise, the rate of IHD falls a bit, then goes up a bit. Nothing very dramatic. But for women, as cholesterol levels got higher, the rate of death from IHD fell by 40 per cent and pretty much stayed there, even when the total cholesterol level was above 7.0mmol/l.[7]

This was a long-term study done on people living in a single country, and it showed that ... Well, I don't really need to tell you. It is, as they say, bleeding obvious. The interesting thing is that it does appear that women do significantly better with higher levels. For men, the cholesterol level is pretty much unimportant, at least when it comes to IHD.

This protective effect of higher cholesterol has also been seen in Japan. In the Jichi Medical School Cohort Study there were no deaths from MI in women with the highest cholesterol levels > 6.21mmol/l. This was a study lasting12 years, and there were 7,500 women in this group. And not one single death from a heart attack.[8]

What the Japanese researchers also noted was that men, in the lowest cholesterol group, had a 50 per cent increase in overall mortality. Women in the lowest cholesterol group also had a 50 per cent increase in overall mortality. The conclusions of the study were that: 'Low cholesterol was related to high mortality even after excluding deaths due to liver disease from the analysis. High cholesterol was not a risk factor for mortality.'

Another squadron of black elephants lumbers overhead, blotting out the sun.

I hasten to add that these are far from isolated studies, they are not outliers. It is the simplest thing in the world to find research and facts that flatly contradict the cholesterol hypothesis. They come from everywhere, every country, all populations.

Not long ago I agreed to co-author a paper looking at all the research that measured LDL levels, and the association with overall mortality. This was in the elderly (i.e. over 60, which I now think of as middle aged). We used the term LDL-C in this paper (which is basically LDL/cholesterol, which is basically LDL).

It was published in the *British Medical Journal Open*. (*Open* means free to view.) At the risk of self-aggrandisement, it was also the most read paper in the journal for five months in a row. We found that: '*High LDL-C is inversely associated with mortality* in most people over 60 years. This finding is inconsistent with the cholesterol hypothesis (i.e., that cholesterol, particularly LDL-C, is inherently atherogenic). Since elderly people with high LDL-C live as long or longer than those with low LDL-C, our analysis provides reason to question the validity of the cholesterol hypothesis.'[9]

Let me translate. In older people, the higher your LDL level, the longer you will live. Of course, it was immediately attacked from all sides. You can see the British Heart Foundation take on it here – https://www.bhf.org. uk/heart-matters-magazine/news/behind-the-headlines/ cholesterol-and-statins. The main attacker was Professor Colin Baigent, from Oxford, who is a leading light in the Clinical Trials Research Unit. The CTRU's home page states that 'It is funded by the Medical Research Council, British Heart Foundation Cancer Research UK, other charities, governmental organisations and pharmaceutical companies.'

The main gist of Professor Baigent's argument is that lowering cholesterol with statins reduces the risk of CVD and death, which proves that a high cholesterol level must be deadly and should be lowered. As I have pointed out, no, it does not. It is clear that statins have many different effects and do not work by lowering LDL; their benefits are due to a positive impact on nitric oxide synthesis. LDL lowering is an unfortunate side effect.

It also needs to be pointed out that PCSK9 inhibitors also lower LDL to a greater degree than statins, yet they were shown to increase the risk of overall, and CV, mortality. Which kind of strengthens our argument and kicks his into touch.

What else, where else to go? I could keep quoting contradictory facts until I'm blue in the face, but it would get somewhat tedious. Thus, I am only going to do five more:

- The Framingham Study
- The Austrian Study
- The (other) American study
- The Worldwide Study
- The hidden studies

THE FRAMINGHAM STUDY

Framingham is a town near Boston in the US. Researchers decided to use the people living there for a long-term study in an attempt identify the factors that are associated with CVD. All adults who agreed to participate became subjects, and had their height, weight, blood pressure, cholesterol levels, food consumption, etc., monitored. It started in 1948 and continues today, which means it even outdates BBC radio's *The Archers*.

Framingham is where it was first decreed or demonstrated – some say proved – that a raised cholesterol level causes CVD. The effect was not gigantic, but it existed, and lo the cholesterol hypothesis was born. Actually, this is not quite true ... And lo, the cholesterol hypothesis was given a massive boost.

It is certainly true that in Framingham the following statement *was* born, and has been repeated endlessly. 'The results of the Framingham study indicate that a 1 per cent reduction in cholesterol corresponds to a 2 per cent reduction in CHD risk.' This idea first appeared in the AHA-NIH publication *The Cholesterol Facts*. This '1 per cent, 2 per cent' statement has gone on to gain the status of inarguable fact.

Now, the best thing about the Framingham Study is that it just keeps churning on and on, which means that we can see what happens to people over extended periods, something that shines light upon complex questions. And lo, in 1987 researchers went back to look at what happened to people in Framingham if their cholesterol levels started to fall. Presumably a 1 per cent fall would lead to a 2 per cent drop in the risk of CHD.

Not quite. Here is what they found: 'There is a direct association between falling cholesterol levels over the first fourteen years (of the study) and mortality over the following eighteen years.' That association, however, was not in the expected direction.

For every 1mg/dl fall in cholesterol (0.026mmol/l), there was an 11 per cent increase in overall mortality, and a 14 per cent increase in CVD deaths.[10] Roughly, this means that a 1 per cent fall in cholesterol level results in a 25 per cent increase in overall mortality, and a 30 per cent increase in CVD death. At one time I would have been surprised, even shocked, that researches into heart disease can say something that can be so perfectly contradicted by their own evidence.

Such matters have now become wearisomely familiar to me. Stated facts are not slightly inaccurate or moderately biased, they are simply twisted round through 180 degrees, then hammered to the wall and presented as the truth.

'You are a slow learner, Winston.'
'How can I help it? How can I help but see what is
in front of my eyes? Two and two are four.'
'Sometimes, Winston. Sometimes they are five.
Sometimes they are three. Sometimes they are all of
them at once. You must try harder. It is not easy to
become sane.'
(George Orwell, *1984*)

THE AUSTRIAN STUDY

In total numbers, the biggest study that I am aware of comes from Austria. I am going to give you the exact figures because they were big. In this study, 67,413 men and 82,237 women (aged 20–95 years) underwent 454,448 tests. These included measurement of blood pressure, height, weight, fasting samples for cholesterol and a few other things. It lasted fifteen years, from 1985–99.

So, what did they find? First, with regard to overall mortality: 'The relationship between low cholesterol level and all-cause mortality is confirmed for both men and women of < 50 years. This contradicts previous assessments that low cholesterol level is just a proxy or marker for frailty occurring with age.'

Translation. Those under 50 with lower cholesterol levels had an increased risk of death over the 15 years of the study. And what of the entire population? 'In men, across the entire age range, although of borderline significance under the age of 50, and in women from the age of 50 onward only, low cholesterol was significantly associated with all-cause mortality, showing significant associations with death through cancer, liver diseases, and mental diseases.'[11]

As always, the meaning of this study is not made clear. Saying that 'low cholesterol was significantly associated with all-cause mortality' could mean lower, or higher, all-cause mortality. You read this stuff and you think, what the bloody hell are they saying? I suppose it is deliberate.

What they really meant to say was that low cholesterol was significantly associated with *higher* all-cause mortality. There, how difficult was that. Add one word and all becomes clear. Were they having trouble with the word count? If so, it was a strange choice to get rid of the single most important word in the study.

One thing they did find was that, in men but not women, higher blood cholesterol levels were associated with a higher risk of CVD. However, I am going to turn this around by utilising the world-famous Dr Kendrick conjecture, most simply written as 'you can only die of one thing'. If more people with *low* cholesterol die of cancer and liver diseases and mental diseases, they cannot then die of CVD. Thus, as more people die of other things, the overall rate of CVD deaths in that population will appear to fall. On the other hand, if more people with high cholesterol do not die of cancer and liver disease and mental disease they are then more likely to die from CVD. Yes, you have to die from something.

I have previously used the analogy of throwing people off high cliffs. If you throw people off high cliffs, everyone will die of severe impact injuries, and no one will die from CVD. Thus, you could reduce the rate of CVD deaths to zero by killing everybody before they have a chance to die of a heart attack or stroke. But what have you proved? That throwing people off cliffs prevents all CVD deaths and therefore should be used as a preventative strategy? I would argue that this is not the most appropriate conclusion.

This 'you can only die of one thing' conjecture is the reason why I emphasise the overall mortality rate as the most important thing to look for in any study or clinical trial. Not the figures on specific causes of mortality. If, for example, you reduce the rate of deaths from heart disease, this is of no benefit to man or beast if people are simply dropping dead of other things at a higher rate. All you have changed is what is written on the death certificate.

Anyway, what the Austrian study – 'Why Eve Is Not Adam: Prospective Follow-Up in 149,650 Women and Men of Cholesterol and Other Risk Factors Related to Cardiovascular and All-Cause Mortality' – demonstrated is that if you have a lower cholesterol level you are more likely to die young. And, of course, vice versa.

THE (OTHER) AMERICAN STUDY

Looking at things from a different perspective, if a high cholesterol level causes CHD then you would expect that people admitted to hospital with MIs would have higher than average levels of cholesterol, would you not? The correct answer to this question is, yes you would.

In 2009, a group of researchers in the US looked at the data from 231,986 hospitalisations with heart attacks, gathered from over 500 hospitals. Cholesterol levels were documented in 136,905 individuals, which is probably enough to be getting on with. Now, in 2009, the mean LDL level in the US was 105mg/dl(2.6mmol/l).[12] In this US study, the mean LDL level of the 136,905 patients admitted to hospital with MI was 104.9mg/dl (2.6mmol/l).[13] I would imagine that, if the average height of everyone in the US was 1.67m, then the average height of those admitted to hospital with MI was also 1.67m. Which is what you would except as height has nothing to do with MIs either.

THE WORLDWIDE STUDY

A couple of years ago Dr Zoe Harcombe, a fellow cholesterol sceptic, decided to look at the cholesterol levels in all the countries in the world, as gathered by the WHO, i.e. all countries where the levels had been measured anyway, plotting this against both CVD deaths and overall mortality. For the sake of brevity I am sticking with overall mortality.

CVD deaths & cholesterol

WHO data for CVD rates vs cholesterol (females)

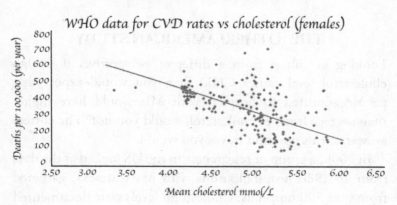

WHO data for CVD rates vs cholesterol (males)

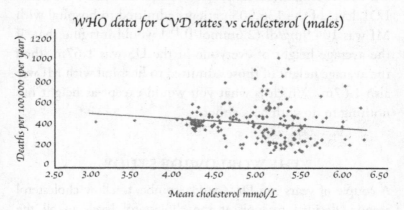

THE HIDDEN STUDIES

Again, we would all like to believe that research is a pure and lofty Olympian ideal. If we cannot trust those involved in medical research to achieve even a basic level of honesty, then what?

Whilst falsifying results is always a possibility and extremely difficult to spot, the greatest difficulty is not with biased studies, it is with findings that are simply not published. As with the research on anti-depressants, if we can see only the trials that were 'successful' whilst everything else is buried, our knowledge will be irredeemably skewed in one direction or another.

And this leads us to two dietary studies where researchers replaced saturated fatty acids with polyunsaturated fatty acids. The first was the Sydney Diet Heart Study, from 1966–73, a time, it should be added, before the dietary guidelines stated that there was no evidence that reducing saturated fats could do any harm.

At the end of the study, the data was not fully published. Critically, deaths due to CVD and CHD were not reported. Luckily, all was not lost because another group of researchers did manage to get hold of the original trial data. They reanalysed it and concluded: 'In this cohort, substituting dietary n-6 LA (Omega 6 linoleic acid) in place of SFA [saturated fatty acids] increased the risks of death from all causes, coronary heart disease, and cardiovascular disease ... These findings could have important implications for worldwide dietary advice to substitute n-6 LA, or PUFAs [polyunsaturated fatty acids] in general, for SFA.'[14]

In this reanalysed study, they discovered that if you replaced saturated fatty acids with super-healthy polyunsaturated fats, you increased the rate of death from CVD and overall mortality. What they did not say, but what needs to be said, is that those writing the dietary guidelines were effectively lied to. Here was research showing that polyunsaturated fatty acids are damaging rather than protective, but it was hidden. Which, in turn, takes us to the Minnesota Coronary Experiment (MCE Trial). This was a far bigger study on the effect of replacing saturated fatty acids with polyunsaturated fatty acids. Indeed, it was biggest ever done. It too was carried out from 1968–73 but, unlike the Sydney Diet Heart Study, no results were published – at all. It was completely buried.

Luckily, the same group of researchers that reviewed the Sydney Study managed to find the original data for the MCE. It was still stored in the garage of the son of one the main researchers.[15] When they reviewed it, far more interesting data emerged. Those who ate the high polyunsaturated fatty acid diet did see a significant drop in cholesterol levels, of around 13 per cent. Hoorah. However, for every 0.78mmol/l reduction in cholesterol, there was a 22 per cent increased risk of death. To repeat, the more the cholesterol level fell, the greater the increased risk of death.[16]

Yes, here we have another study demonstrating that replacing saturated fatty acids with the polyunsaturated kind was not just useless, but damaging. Once again, this fact could have been presented to those writing the guidelines in the late 1970s, but it was not. It was hidden away in a garage.

At which point, I would like to ask thee quick questions. Can you possibly imagine who was the driving force, the lead researcher on the MCE? Who, almost single-handedly, was responsible for driving the diet-heart hypothesis in the first place? The man who destroyed John Yudkin for daring to suggest that sugar may be more damaging than saturated fatty acids?

Yes, it was he who cannot be named ... Ancel Keys.

THOSE WITH FH ARE FAR MORE LIKELY TO DIE OF CVD, AND AT A YOUNG AGE

I think I have dealt with the 'statins lower LDL and reduce the risk of CVD' argument. So, I will move straight on to the FH argument. Here is the lair of the beast, the fortress, the adamantine core of the thing. Whenever they seem to be in danger of losing the argument that LDL causes CVD, those who promote the LDL hypothesis will retreat here and bellow from the ramparts:

'People with FH die young from CVD, which means that high LDL level must be the cause of CVD!'

The first thing to consider with FH is the following. It is caused by having a lack of, or improperly functioning, LDL receptors. It can be heterozygous (a defective LDL gene from one parent) or homozygous (genes from both parents). In heterozygous FH the LDL level will be at least twice 'normal', say around 7.5mmol/l up to about 13mmol/l. In homozygous it can be anything above 20mmol/l up to 50mmol/l.

What does this tell us? Well, that without LDL receptors to remove it, LDL remains trapped in the bloodstream. Ponder that thought for a moment – *in the bloodstream*. Why is it not simply leaking through artery walls to escape and cause plaques? The answer is because it cannot leak through. Also note that a lack of LDL receptors means cells are starved of vital, life-enhancing cholesterol. Do you think this might cause problems? If so, consider the fact that any harm caused by FH may be due to sub-optimal cholesterol in all cells in the body, rather than high cholesterol in the blood. Just a thought.

However, to get back to the more straightforward arguments about FH. It is widely accepted, even by me, that the risk of CVD (only CHD, not a stroke) is greatly increased in FH. Various statistics are thrown about with gay abandon, but it is commonly stated that younger people with FH are four or five times more likely to die from CHD than anyone else. Superficially, this seems inarguable proof that very high LDL truly does cause CHD. However …

The first thing to say is that younger people are very unlikely to die from CHD in the first place. Whilst the four to five times figure is often quoted, it needs to be borne in mind that this statistic is for twenty-to thirty-year-olds where increasing the risk by 400 per cent, in absolute terms, is far less dramatic than you might think.

In general, people aged twenty to thirty have about one-hundredth the rate of death from CHD of those sixty-four and above. So, if you increase the risk of death in this group, it will have an almost indiscernible effect on overall CVD mortality. This is not meant to come across as heartless, it is just a fact.[17]

In absolute terms, if you quadrupled the rate of CHD in women aged twenty to thirty, this would increase CHD deaths by around 0.5 per thousand per year. If you quadrupled the rate in women above sixty-four, this would result in an increase of 100 extra deaths per 1,000 per year. So, you can state that FH vastly increases the risk of CHD by as much as 400 or 500 per cent, and if this sounds incredibly dramatic, it is meant to. The reality is that the absolute impact on CHD risk is extremely small. It is the old relative v absolute risk game again. As a wise man once said: 'Figures don't lie, but liars sure know how to figure.'

Another fact that needs to be highlighted is that the impact of FH lessens considerably, then disappears, as people get older. 'In summary, treated FH was associated with a substantial excess mortality from CHD in young adults, but no significant excess was found in patients aged 60 or more.'[18]

I now want you to ponder this a little more deeply. Here is a condition that increases the death rate from CHD, in younger people, but has no impact on older people. Try replacing the words FH and CHD with smoking and lung cancer, and then try this statement. Young people who smoke are far more likely to die from lung cancer, but after the age of sixty smoking has no effect on lung cancer. So, after sixty, just keep on smoking.

If this were true, would it not make you question that fact that smoking does cause cancer? Of course, the 'healthy survivor' argument is used. Namely, those who were going to die of FH died young, leaving healthy survivors. Having FH is the very condition that is supposed to make you unhealthy in the first place. How can there be any healthy survivors? This argument self-destructs on contact with logic.

Another major problem with the entire 'FH is deadly' argument emerged as early as 1966, when it was found that people with FH lived just as long as everyone else. 'Our studies provide no evidence that familial hypercholesterolemia appreciably shortens the life of affect individuals, either male or female. On the contrary, they show that high levels of serum cholesterol are clearly compatible with survival into the seventh and eighth decades.'[19]

Even those running the Simon Broome register (set up to study FH many years ago) must admit that those with

FH actually have a lower overall mortality rate than the surrounding population, despite the much higher rate of heart disease. 'Importantly, in patients without known coronary disease at registration (with the Simon Broome registry), *all-cause mortality was significantly lower than in the general population*, mainly due to a reduction of more than one-third in the risk of fatal cancer. The data also confirm our earlier findings that FH patients are not at a higher risk of fatal stroke.'[20]

FH is indeed a terrible disease. It causes no symptoms, you are far less likely to die from cancer and you live longer than anyone else. OMG! We must treat it as aggressively as possible.

At which point, I would like to return to the issue of strokes. Strangely, and almost unremarked upon by anyone, anywhere – in fact I will guarantee that you have never heard of it – is the fact that a raised LDL is *not* a risk factor for a stroke, neither in the normal population nor the FH population. And that's despite the fact that the clear majority of strokes are caused by atherosclerotic plaques developing in the carotid arteries, which is the exact same underlying cause for most MIs.

A massive study published in *The Lancet* over twenty years ago looked at nearly half a million people to try and find an association between strokes and raised blood cholesterol, but no such association could be found.[21]

Even in FH, LDL is not a risk factor for a stroke, yet lowering LDL with statins still reduces the risk? Indeed, if you have had a stroke you will be virtually forced to take statins. I have raised this issue on-line, in debates and in discussions with cardiologists. They just look at me blankly. Perhaps you can phrase this better than me: 'Raised LDL is not a risk factor for a stroke, even in FH. However, lowering LDL with statins reduces the risk of a stroke. Could you please explain how this can be? Unless, the benefit of statins has nothing to do with LDL lowering?'

I find it quite amazing that no one else seems remotely bothered by the problems for the LDL/cholesterol hypothesis raised by this conundrum, whereas I consider it of key importance. Maybe I am missing something.

Another surprising fact about FH is that the actual level of LDL has no effect on risk. 'There was an up to 5-fold increased risk of CHD hazards in the familial hypercholesterolemia phenotype group for the index age of 20 to 29 years. Conversely, there were relatively lower hazards at older ages, particularly a nonsignificant increase in risk between 70 to 79 years of age. Interestingly, there was also *no significant interaction between races (black and nonblack) and LDL-C levels on the hazard ratios.*'[22]

Isaac Asimov said: 'The most exciting phrase in science, the one that heralds most discoveries, is not "Eureka!" but "That's funny".' And it is funny that everyone with FH will have very high LDL levels, but some will have far higher levels than others, up to three times as high. However, the level itself bears no relationship to the risk of heart disease, and this has been noted in many studies on heterozygous FH, where this has been looked at.

At least, it's funny if you have an ounce of curiosity in your soul. How can it possibly be that having FH increases your risk of heart disease, but the actual level of LDL in those with FH is irrelevant? You can chase this one around as much as you like, but in the end once you stop squirming there can be only one answer. There is something else going on, something that connects CHD to FH.

In classic epidemiology this is often explained using the 'yellow fingers/lung cancer association'. People with yellow fingers are more likely to die of lung cancer. So, yellow fingers cause lung cancer? No, smoking causes both yellow fingers and lung cancer. But what underlying factor could possibly cause both FH and an increased risk of CHD? Well, you may have noticed a theme emerging in this book: blood clotting has a major part to play in CVD, not just in causing the final event but all the way through the development of atherosclerosis. Could it be possible that blood clotting and FH are related in some way? Why, I'm glad you asked.

The first time I spotted the importance of clotting factors was way back in the 1980s with the publication of the Scottish Heart Study, where a raised fibrinogen was found to be a very potent risk factor for CVD. Then, more relevantly, I stumbled over a paper from 1985 looking at people with FH who did, and who did not, have diagnosed CHD.

'Haemostatic variables (clotting variables) were measured in 61 patients with heterozygous FH, 32 of whom had had evidence of coronary heart disease. Age adjusted means concentrations of *plasma fibrinogen and factor VIII were significantly higher* in these patients than in the 29 patients without coronary heart disease, but there were *no significant differences in serum lipid concentrations between the two groups.*'[23]

Half the people with FH had CHD, and the other half did not. The difference between them was that the levels of fibrinogen and factor VIII were significantly higher in those with CHD. The other thing I want to highlight here, which was passed over in this paper without comment, is that in almost half of the FH patients there was *no* evidence of CVD. Surely not. That's interesting ... but not, I suppose, if you lack the desire to be interested.

The fact is that if you choose to look at FH from a different perspective, it becomes clear that FH, alone, does not increase the risk of CHD. You must also have some form of blood clotting abnormality. As it turns out, these are far more common in people with FH. 'Platelet-dependent thrombin generation was increased in patients with hypercholesterolemia, indicating that *hypercholesterolemia is associated with hypercoagulability* through the interaction between platelets and coagulation factors.'[24]

In addition to all this, there are some highly complex interactions between the LDL receptor itself and factor VIII, which leads to a reduced clearance of factor VIII and therefore increased risk of blood clotting. Finally, in an attempt to close the loop here, it has been found that statins have a significant effect on blood clotting in FH patients: 'Statins, the well-known lipid-lowing drugs not only decrease blood lipid levels but also reduce coagulation activity through the downregulation of tissue factor [TF] in blood monocyte and endothelial cells. Moreover, *long-term statin treatment can reduce coagulation activity in subjects with hypercholesterolemia.* In the same way, our data imply an association of hyperlipidemia with hypercoagulability.'[25]

Indeed, wherever you look in both CVD and FH, you end up staring straight at blood clotting. This is especially true in FH where a raised LDL, and an increased risk of blood clotting, are intimately related.

I could go on, but I shall stop here as I am acutely aware that I have been getting highly technical at times and many find this too much. So, let's finish by reiterating that, yes, there is a clear association between FH and CHD (in some, but not in all people). However, the connection between the two is not directly causal. There are just too many contradictions.

- The level of LDL in FH is not related to the risk of CHD
- FH is not associated with an increase in stroke risk
- FH only increases the risk of CHD in a younger population, not in the age group where CHD is far more likely to kill you
- FH only increases the risk of CHD if you also have some form of thrombophilia (increased blood clotting tendency)

CHAPTER 14

How to Avoid Dying of CVD and Anything Else

In my first book, *The Great Cholesterol Con*, I covered the issues of how to avoid dying of CVD in about half a paragraph. I did this on the basis that the last thing the world needed was more health advice. However, a few people suggested to me very politely that I was a COMPLETE IDIOT. People want to know what to DO. I think that might have been my sister. She was not alone.

So, I am going to delve a bit deeper and give my 'Ten steps to avoid heart disease'. In truth, I have no idea if there are ten steps or not, but it sounds about right. Actually, before starting, I shall rename this my 'Ten steps to living longer', as most of what is good for CVD is also good for overall health.

First, though, I also want to give you some idea of the absolute scale of risk and benefit we are talking about because I do not want to blow small differences out of proportion. Whilst I have banged on about such things as excess carbohydrate intake increasing the risk of obesity, and diabetes and CVD, etc., these do not represent massive risks.

I hope I managed to make it clear that figures can be inflated out of all proportion. For example, a claimed 36 per cent reduction in CHD shrivels down to virtually nothing on closer inspection. The same is true of most other studies, especially the dietary ones. Here the experts battle over the most minute reduction and increases in risk, so small that they could simply be artefacts. A couple of extra tosses of the coin coming up heads.

If you used Sigma 5 to determine the success of a trial, you would find that there would be almost no evidence left to look at. My own view is that, unless you can see at least a doubling, or halving of risk, the effect is best ignored. Or, to put this another way, I really am not interested in say hazard ratios of 1.12 (a 12 per cent increase in risk): 12 per cent of bugger-all is still, pretty much, bugger-all. I want to see some truly significant impact on life expectancy.

At present, the moment an observational study manages to squeak past the hallowed p <0.05, it ends up as a newspaper headline, like 'Coffee Will Save Your Life'. Hold on a minute, it kills you, no – it's good for you, no – bad ... aaarrrggghhh. Currently, the evidence seems to be that it is probably good for you. Well, drink coffee if you want, but I wouldn't be too bothered about the effect on health, one way or another.

Returning to statins, they have been repeatedly hailed as the wonder drug of all wonder drugs. In reality, they increase life expectancy by about three to four days after five years of treatment. This means that, if you took them for thirty years, assuming the benefits are real, you might get about a month extra on the planet. Trade that off against thirty years of muscle pain and weakness, loss of libido, brain fog, etc. I suspect you could probably live longer if you were put in an induced coma, fed through a tube and suspended by wires from the ceiling. However, any increase in life expectancy needs to be balanced against squeezing a few scraps of enjoyment out of life.

As for blood pressure lowering tablets. Well, if you have very high blood pressure, they might give you around an extra month as well. What about lowering blood sugar levels in diabetes. It seems that if you try too hard to get sugar levels back to 'normal' this may well actually reduce life expectancy. As mentioned before, the lower you get the blood sugar, the greater the risk of early death.[1]

What if you take lots and lots of tablets at the same time, to decrease the risk of heart disease, stroke, diabetes and anything else you can think of, a strategy known as polypharmacy. Do the benefits multiply together to create one big, happy, life-extending medical smorgasbord of medication?

This is hard to say, for sure, and the data is extremely difficult to analyse. However, it seems that if you are reasonably healthy and you take lots of drugs this will decrease, rather than increase, your life expectancy.[2] If you are frail and taking lots of drugs, things get even worse, as this will vastly increase your risk of early death by over 500 per cent (relative risk).[3]

If you have multimorbidity, suffering from several different diagnosed diseases at the same time, e.g. heart disease, heart failure, AF, chronic obstructive pulmonary disease, diabetes, etc., then taking a whole whack of different medications may be beneficial. This makes sense. And if you have many different diseases, you will be taking a whole set of different drugs for a reason – hopefully. For example, diuretics to reduce fluid overload, and take pressure off the heart, in heart failure. Also warfarin to prevent strokes in AF, and ACE-inhibitors to protect the heart after MI. These are most definitely individually beneficial, and should add to together to create greater overall benefit, which you could equate as benefit > harm.

The evidence does appear to show that taking multiple medications to treat multiple specific problems is a good idea, even if you take a lot of different drugs. Even so, we need to be far more careful in the frail elderly as the harm/ benefit equation shifts to harm.

However, do not rely on 'preventive' polypharmacy to stop diseases happening. This strategy simply does not work. In my opinion, the damage caused by polypharmacy is almost certainly the major reason why life expectancy is currently falling in the elderly in the UK.[4]

Before getting too side-tracked, though, I shall leave aside the small players here and turn to the big-ticket items that can shorten your lifespan – by years. And here they are:

- Smoking
- Lack of exercise
- Avoiding sunshine
- Poor social interactions/mental stress

The dangers of smoking are well established and non-controversial. I have seen different figures but, if you smoke 20 a day, you will reduce your lifespan by around six years. If you smoke 40 a day, that's eight to ten years. And both give all sorts of unpleasant, long-term health consequences. Once you have seen your 10,000th patient gasping for breath, unable to walk, coughing their guts up with a cyborg plastic tube linking them to oxygen cylinders, you tend to take a pretty dim view of smoking. At least I do.

With exercise, the figures are a bit more all over the place. However, a recent, very large study came to the following conclusions about the impact on life expectancy of exercise v remaining sedentary:

- 75 minutes of brisk walking per week equates to an extra 1.8 years of life expectancy
- 150–299 minutes of brisk walking per week and the gain in life expectancy goes up to 3.4 years.
- 450 minutes per week and the estimated life expectancy increases by 4.5 years[5]

The caveat here is that people taking a lot of exercise tend to follow other healthy lifestyles, i.e.. they don't smoke or drink to excess and have a positive mental attitude. Disentangling one positive factor from another is always tricky, however much the researchers may claim to have done so.

Having said this, I know what you are thinking, because I was thinking it too – 450 minutes *a week*. That is slightly more than an hour a day, which is mega. I think I am quite good on the exercise front, but I average about half an hour a day, max. Still, them's the figures, so disagree with them if you will. Note to self: 'Am I happy to lounge about a bit and shorten my life by a year? Answer ... probably. One hour of reasonably intense exercise a day ... that makes me tired just thinking about it.

Anyway, what we know so far is that if you don't smoke, and spend 450 minutes a week exercising, this will give you around ten and a half extra, healthy years on this planet. Not bad. I heartily recommend them both, even if I will almost certainly fail to do the required exercise.

You may have noted that the first two items on my list are very much in line with mainstream advice. Nothing very startling here at all. The next two may be a little more controversial. The first is something I have not mentioned up to now because it didn't really fit in. Sunshine is exceedingly healthy and exceedingly good for you, and increased exposure to the sun will mean that you live far longer.

Yes, I know, we are all screamed at on a regular basis to avoid any risk that a few stray photons may dare to brush against your skin. This will cause skin cancer, and YOU WILL DIE. And it will be ALL YOUR OWN FAULT. Ho hum, fiddle-dee-dee. Get stuffed.

Do you know why Caucasians are pale and uninteresting? It is because if you have dark skin and live a long way from the equator, the sun cannot produce enough vitamin D on contact with your skin. So, those of us who migrated northwards, especially the Scots, went white lest we become vitamin D deficient and die. Then we developed ginger hair, although I have no idea why that happened. One of nature's jokes. I blame the Neanderthals.

My general view on sunshine is very simple. We evolved to live out in the open, under the sun. It would seem unimaginably weird if it turned out that the sun is inimical to life. Most animals, and we too are animals, evolved to be outside all day, every day, come rain or shine.

Therefore, it seems basic evolutionary logic to propose that avoiding the sun might represent unhealthy rather than healthy behaviour. Our skin did not turn pale so that we could hide in a cave all day.

For many years I had been unearthing evidence that avoiding sunshine was not a great health strategy, but my thinking crystallised with some force in 2009 when I came across a paper in the *Annals of Epidemiology* called 'Vitamin D for cancer prevention: Global perspective.' This paper contained some extraordinary results:

- Women with higher UVB exposure had only half the rate of breast cancer
- Men with higher UVB exposure had only half the rate of fatal prostate cancer
- Men and women with higher vitamin D levels had one quarter the risk of developing colon cancer.[6]

Blimey, I thought, greater exposure to sunshine more than halves the rate of three of the most common cancers there are. But, I hear you cry, what about skin cancer?

First, it should be pointed out that there are several different types of skin cancer, and whilst no one wants cancer, most skin cancers can be quickly diagnosed and fully cured. The three common ones are: basal cell carcinoma (BCC), squamous cell carcinoma (SCC) and rodent ulcers. These are sometimes grouped together as non-melanoma cancers.

There seems little doubt that the non-melanoma skin cancers are caused by excess sun exposure, particularly on pale-skinned people who live in countries (e.g. South Africa, Australia, California and Hong Kong) closer to the equator than their skin was designed for. Indeed, having looked at the mangled and scarred scalps of some elderly ex-pats, I would most definitely recommend hats for sun protection, at the very least. You don't want to spend your later years having nasty things scraped off your head every six months.

As for using sun cream, things are far more contentious. There is a strong argument to be made that sun tan lotions can do more harm than good. They stop you burning, yes, but can let through UVA, which may be the truly dangerous form of radiation. It is also possible that the chemicals in sun creams themselves are carcinogenic. Personally, I would recommend gradually building up a tan and using as little sunscreen as possible. If you do use sun cream, I would strongly recommend a sun cream that blocks both UVB and UVA.

What then of malignant melanoma? We have been repeatedly informed, with ever-increasing levels of hysteria, that this, the deadliest form of skin cancer, is increasing dramatically year on year. And that this is all due to excess sun exposure. Is this actually true? Well, probably not.

In my medical career I was taught that if an agent is to be considered a true cause of a disease, it must have been present, at some point. For example, if you came across people suffering from TB, in whom you could find no trace of the tuberculous bacillus (past or present), you would be unable to claim it was *the* agent that caused TB.

Now malignant melanomas can be found in several different places where the sun does not shine, at all. The mother of a friend of mine died of melanoma that started in the inner lining of her nose. Melanomas can also develop in the oesophagus and the vagina. In short, sunlight is *not* required for malignant melanomas to develop. In addition, it has long been known that melanomas are far less likely to develop in those who work outdoors, as noted in an article in *The Lancet*: 'Outdoor workers have a decreased risk of melanoma compared with indoor workers, suggesting that chronic sunlight exposure can have a protective effect. Further, some melanomas form on sun-exposed regions; others do not ... It has long been realised that indoor workers have an increased risk for melanoma compared with those who work outdoors, suggesting that ultraviolet radiation is in some way protective against this (melanoma) cancer. Further, melanoma develops most often on the back of men and on the legs of women, areas that are not chronically exposed to the sun.'[7]

Another 'that's funny' fact is that the diagnosed rate of malignant melanomas has continued to rise, even though people really and truly have been scared witless of the sun. Many people now hide from it, cover up and slap on factor 50 sun cream at the slightest hint of light. This suggests that something else may be going on. Greater recognition of early, non-serious melanomas, perhaps? A study in the UK concluded that there has been no true rise. It is publicity, fear and misdiagnosis that has created the apparent epidemic of melanoma. The article in the *British Journal of Dermatology*, entitled 'Melanoma epidemic: a midsummer night's dream?', concluded: 'the large increase in reported incidence is likely to be due to diagnostic drift which classifies benign lesions as stage one melanoma ... The distribution of the lesions (melanomas) reported did not correspond to the sites of lesions caused by solar exposure. These findings should lead to a reconsideration of the treatment of 'early' lesions, a search for better diagnostic methods to distinguish them from truly malignant melanomas, re-evaluation of the role of ultraviolet radiation and recommendations for protection from it, as well as the need for a new direction in the search for the cause of melanoma.'[8]

Yes, despite what you have heard, the evidence that sun exposure is the cause of malignant melanomas is patchy, inconsistent and often flatly contradicted by the facts. It could actually be more strongly argued that sun exposure may reduce, rather than increase, the risk of melanoma. For example, a study in the US looked at people who had previously been diagnosed with melanoma to establish the impact of further sun exposure on the risk of subsequent melanoma development and survival. It said: 'Sunburn, high intermittent sun exposure, skin awareness histories, and solar elastosis were statistically significantly inversely associated with death from melanoma' and concluded, 'Sun exposure is associated with increased survival from melanoma.'[9] Why? Probably because one of the main effects of sunlight on the skin is to create vitamin D, and vitamin D has been found to have very powerful anti-cancer effects.[10]

However, it is not only vitamin D that is increased by sun exposure because it has recently been discovered that sunlight greatly increases NO (as in nitric oxide) synthesis.[11] Yes, my favourite chemical for CV health.

It appears that this increase in NO also directly translates into a significant CV benefit. There have been a series of studies from Sweden and Denmark that have looked at women who sunbathe regularly vs those who avoid the sun. They have all found the same thing. A significant reduction in CV death and a significant increase in life expectancy in the sun-lovers. One of the most recent of these papers even concluded that sun avoidance was as bad for health as smoking.

Nonsmokers who avoided sun exposure had a life expectancy similar to smokers in the highest sun exposure group, indicating that avoidance of *sun exposure is a risk factor for death of a similar magnitude as smoking*. Compared to the highest sun exposure group, life expectancy of avoiders of sun exposure was reduced by 0.6-2.1 years.'[12]

This was a twenty-year study. If average life expectancy is around eighty years, we can safely multiply those figures by four to work out that a decent amount of sun exposure can add from three to eight years to your life expectancy. And at this point I am happy to stick my neck on the block and to state that I believe the official advice to avoid the sun, and never go outside without liberally slapping on sun cream, has been the single most damaging piece of preventive medical advice in history. There have been other stupid things, that it true, but this stands out as *the* most stupid and *the* most damaging. Which, it must be added, takes some doing in such a strong field of contenders.

Here, for your perusal, is a more complete list of benefits of increased sun exposure that have been uncovered. I am giving you the most positive figures:

- Colorectal cancer 75 per cent reduction
- Breast cancer 50 per cent reduction
- Non-Hodgkin's lymphoma 20–40 per cent reduction[13]
- Prostate cancer 50 per cent reduction
- Bladder cancer 30 per cent reduction
- Metabolic syndrome/type 2 diabetes 40 per cent reduction
- Alzheimer's 50 per cent reduction
- Multiple sclerosis 50 per cent reduction
- Psoriasis 60 per cent reduction
- Macular degeneration seven-fold reduction in risk
- Improvement in mood/wellbeing[14]

There is almost nothing that is better for you than sun exposure. Not only that, it is free and enjoyable. Who could ask for anything more? And just one more thing, this quote: 'Sunlight Has Cardiovascular Benefits Independently of Vitamin D'. 'All-cause mortality should be the primary determinant of public health messages. Sunlight is a risk factor for skin cancer, but sun avoidance may carry more of a cost than benefit for overall good health.'[15] Quite.

The final big-ticket item on my list is ... poor social interactions and the strain caused by them, or whatever you want to call this rather hard-to-define area. The range of different, interconnected, issues includes: childhood abuse, family breakup, abusive partner, financial difficulties, an abusive and bullying boss at work, social isolation, mental health issues, loneliness, no sense of being part of a supportive family or group, religious or otherwise.

The simple fact is that we humans are social animals. We require nurture and support by others. We need a sense of belonging, a sense of value and purpose. We need to be loved, not hit or shouted at; not bullied or treated with contempt.

When I first started looking at CVD, this was the area that I focused on. It seemed obvious that there was an enormously important mind/body connection that was simply being ignored by mainstream research into heart and all other diseases. Despite the complete lack of interest by most researchers, whenever and wherever you looked, psychological/ mental health issues were standing right there, waving their arms about and shouting me, Me, look at ME.

The full impact of negative stressors was highlighted in a study that was, in a remarkable coincidence, sent to me at the exact moment I was writing this section. Researchers found that people who suffer from significant money worries are 13 times more likely to suffer a heart attack. Yes, 13 times or 1,300 per cent. Now that is the level of increased risk where I tend to prick up my ears and pay attention. Relative risk or not.[16]

It is also clear that mental health, or mental illness, plays a massive role in overall health and life expectancy, as highlighted by researchers from Oxford University. 'Serious mental illnesses reduce life expectancy by 10 to 20 years, an analysis by Oxford University psychiatrists has shown – a loss of years that's equivalent to or worse than that for heavy smoking. The average reduction in life expectancy in people with bipolar disorder is between nine and 20 years, while it is 10 to 20 years for schizophrenia, between nine and 24 years for drug and alcohol abuse, and around seven to 11 years for recurrent depression.'[17]

Yes, when your mind goes wrong, your body follows, with disastrous consequences for overall health. Of course there is an overlap between mental illness, drug use, smoking and suchlike. If you strip out all the other things, you are left with the ferocious power of the mind/body connection; the power to nurture and the power to destroy.

Health, I must emphasise, is a combination of physical, psychological and social wellbeing. Three overlapping sets. The holy trinity. You must get them all right or nothing works. As Plato noted: 'the part can never be well unless the whole is well.'

Who are the shortest-lived peoples in the world? The poor? Not necessarily, although poverty can be a clear cause of ill health. They are those who live in the places of greatest social dislocation and disruption. Or, put another way, those who have had their societies stripped apart. Australian aboriginals, New Zealand Maoris, North American aboriginals and the Inuit.

Indigenous Australians have the worst life expectancy rates of any indigenous population in the world, a United Nations report says. But it's not news to aboriginal health experts. They say it simply confirms what Australian health services have known for years.

Aboriginal Medical Services Alliance of the Northern Territory (AMSANT) chief executive officer John Paterson said the findings of the report, which examined the indigenous populations of 90 countries, were no surprise. The UN report – State of the World's Indigenous Peoples – showed indigenous people in Australia and Nepal fared the worst, dying up to 20 years earlier than their non-indigenous counterparts. In Guatemala, the life expectancy gap is 13 years and in New Zealand it is 11.[18]

The differences in life expectancy in deprived inner-cities in the US and the UK mirror these findings. People do just as badly as Australian aboriginals. It does not take a genius to guess where they might be. Inner-city Glasgow, Manchester, Liverpool and the ghetto areas in virtually all US cities; where the marginalised poor live – but not for terribly long. Do not be a stranger in your own land. It kills you. The differences between places [in the US] are sometimes stark. For example, the average person in San Jose (California District 19) lives to 84 years compared to just 73 years for someone from Kentucky District 5, in the rural south east of that state.'[19]

On a more positive note, living in supporting and positive

environments is exceedingly good for you. The Blue Zones are areas of the world where people live longer than anywhere else, e.g. inland Sardinia, Loma Linda California, Nicoya (Costa Rica), Okinawa, Ikaria (Greece), and a couple of others. I think I should point out that they are also very sunny.

The most important factor was a sense of wellbeing, community, a connection with other people, a sense of purpose and good relationships with friends and family. As a slight aside, the author of the book *The Blue Zones*, Dan Buettner, was very focused on the benefits of a high-vegetable, low-meat diet. He tried hard to promote the idea that diet was the primary driver of good health.

For example, in Sardinia, he wrote the following about the 'typical' diet: 'It's loaded with home-grown fruits and vegetables, such as zucchini, eggplant, tomatoes, and fava beans, that may reduce the risk of heart disease and colon cancer. Also on the table: dairy products, such as milk from grass-fed sheep and pecorino cheese, which, like fish, contribute protein and omega-3 fatty acids.'

The Sardinians however, had a completely different view of what they eat, and they protested at his observations: 'In 2011, Sardinians called for formal recognition of their diet insisting that "the secret to a long life can be found in their traditional diet of lamb, roast piglet, milk and cheese".'[20]

In fact, many years earlier a researcher studied another Italian community that defied all dietary expectations. This was the town of Roseta in Pennsylvania. This community had moved, virtually lock stock and barrel, from Roseta in Italy to a new Roseta in the US. It was noted that they had an extraordinarily low rate of CVD. Why? I quote from the *Huffington Post*:

What made Rosetans die less from heart disease than identical towns elsewhere? Family ties. Another observation: they had traditional and cohesive family and community relationships. It turns out that Roseto was peopled by strongly knit Italian-American families who did everything right and lived right and consequently lived longer.

In short, Rosetans were nourished by people.

In all ways, this happy result was exactly the opposite expectation of well-proven health laws. The Rosetans broke the following long-life rules, and did so with a noticeable relish: and they lived to tell the tale. They smoked old-style Italian stogie cigars, malodorous and remarkably pungent little nips of a cigar guaranteed to give a nicotine fix of unbelievably strong potency. These were not filtered or adulterated in any way.

Both sexes drank wine with seeming abandon, a beverage which the 1963 era dietician would find almost prehistoric in health value. In fact, wine was consumed in preference to all-American soft drinks and even milk. Forget the cushy office job, Rosetan men worked in such toxic environs as the nearby slate quarries. Working there was notoriously dangerous, not merely hazardous, with 'industrial accidents' and gruesome illnesses caused by inhaling gases, dusts and other niceties.

And forget the Mediterranean diets of olive oil, light salads and fat-free foods. No, Rosetans fried their sausages and meatballs in lard. They ate salami, hard and soft cheeses all brimming with cholesterol.[21]

The Okinawans, another of the Blue Zone populations, are also known as pig-eaters. It is said that they eat every part of the pig, apart from the squeak. In short, you can focus on the diet of very long-lived people around the world, if you want, but you will find little or nothing here. And look at the French, with the *highest* consumption of animal fat in Europe and the *lowest* rate of CVD.

Getting back to the main point – The Blue Zones teach us that social health is extremely important. Perhaps the single most important factor of all. If your social health goes wrong, your psychological health will suffer, followed by your physical health. More recently it has been recognised, finally, that loneliness is a significant driver of ill health and early death.[22]

At this point, we have our four big-ticket health items: smoking, lack of exercise, low exposure to sunshine and poor social interactions/health. I did a quick back-of-the-envelope calculation to work out the impact of them on life expectancy. It is not entirely scientific, but I think it is broadly correct.

I made the assumption that we can all live to 100 years old (individual genetics aside). If, that is, we live the optimal lifestyle. Then I included the four factors that will eat away at life expectancy:

- If you smoke 20 a day, you reduce lifespan to 94
- If you smoke and take no exercise, you reduce lifespan to 89
- If you smoke, take no exercise and hide from the sun, you reduce lifespan to 82
- If you smoke, take no exercise, stay out of the sun and have poor social interactions/damaged mental health, you reduce lifespan to 70

Throw in some serious mental illness, and you can get down to 60. Bad luck and bad genetics can lower this even further. You can argue with these figures if you want, but they pretty much reflect what we see in populations around the world.

In short, if you want to live a long and healthy life, these are the four things you should focus on. This is not rocket science, there is no magic pill, alas. I would guess that, apart from sun exposure, you would nod to yourself and agree that you probably knew these things already. Perhaps the absolute impact in years of life expectancy surprised you. Maybe not.

But what of other things. What of diet? This is what most people seem obsessively focused on, to the exclusion of all else. Let's move on.

CHAPTER 15

Diet, Lifespan and CVD

I started my journey of discovery in heart disease far, far, away from diet. Frankly, I wasn't very interested in it. I spent a couple of weeks studying the diet-heart hypothesis at which point it became clear, rapidly, that saturated fat has nothing whatsoever to do with CVD. As far I was concerned that pretty much ended my interest in diet. However, in the last few years I have been dragged back into the dietary battleground with the emergence of the HFLC movement. This idea has been around for many years, but it finally started to gain traction about ten years ago.

As it turned out, most of the people I knew, who agreed with me about diet and cholesterol and statins, etc., were also increasingly vocal supporters of HFLC. They felt that the 'expert' advice on diet, which is to avoid fat and eat carbs, was driving the obesity epidemic, the type 2 diabetes epidemic and thus, indirectly, increasing the risk of CVD.

My initial response was, well everyone in the West is getting fatter and more diabetic and the rate of CVD is still going down. Ergo, there must be something fundamentally wrong with this model. So, I initially resisted the urge to become involved. Then the data began to show that the rate of CVD decline is slowing, even reversing in some countries. Somewhat reluctantly, I delved further.

Having said this, I have always known that the HFLC diet has made perfect physiological sense. The science says that it should be good for you, whereas eating excess carbs could well be bad for you (various provisos apply here). I am not going through the physiology and biochemistry here in any great detail, because that is another book, and there are plenty of books on this topic. I am only going to give you the top line on this, which is ...

If you eat carbohydrates you are eating sugar(s) because all carbs are sugars, and your digestive system will break down all forms of carbohydrate into glucose and fructose. Therefore, after eating carbs, the blood sugar rises. This stimulates insulin release. Insulin, as discussed, drives the conversion of sugar to fat in your liver. In addition, if you keep eating carbs, the insulin level rises to the level where it traps fatty acids in your fat cells, so you cannot release any fat stores (i.e., you get fatter).

Then another bad thing happens. The blood sugar level spikes about an hour after eating, but insulin continues to be released for some time afterwards. This, then, drives the blood sugar down, down below 'normal' causing you to feel very hungry, so you eat again. If you eat carbs the blood sugar rockets back up, followed by insulin. So, your blood sugar level bounds up and down, followed by insulin. Here is my simple, ready reckoner.

Eat carbohydrates → blood sugar rises → insulin rises → blood sugar drops → hungry → eat, rpt: → fat trapped → obesity → type 2 diabetes → CVD

Listen, several people have written books on this, and I just gave it to you in twenty words and nine arrows. This is the nutritional equivalent of $E = MC^2$. But it is true? Can excess carb consumption be *the* health disaster of our age?

Whilst I do not want to go overboard on this, I am increasingly convinced that excess carb consumption is the primary driver of the obesity epidemic, the type 2 diabetes epidemic and that type 2 diabetes is, in turn, a highly significant risk factor for CVD.

What does truly make me angry is the stupid and damaging advice given to people with type 2 diabetes to avoid fat and eat carbs. 'You have trouble controlling your blood sugar level. I have the answer ... eat sugar.' Well, what could possibly go wrong? Just have a look at the statistics on obesity and type 2 diabetes since the dietary advice came into being. Cause and effect.

Nowadays, I strongly advise people who are having trouble with weight gain, verging on obesity, that they must reduce their carb and increase their fat intake. Those with diabetes, absolutely and utterly, must reduce carbs. This is just so obvious that you can only argue against it if you have lost the ability to think. Or if you are on opinion leader in cardiology or diabetes, which is pretty much the same thing.

But what of other dietary fads? There is currently intense promotion of the mythical Mediterranean diet, whatever that might be. I have been to France, Sardinia, Egypt, Croatia, Spain, Israel, Greece and many other countries on the Mediterranean. Frankly, there is bugger-all similarity between their diets. A bit of salad, yes. More fish and olive oil than in Scotland – for sure. Otherwise?

It was Ancel Keys, who else, who started the whole Mediterranean diet thingy, which makes me immediately suspicious. Frankly, if Ancel Keys had said 'I've just discovered the Mediterranean Sea' I'd need to go and dip my toe in it to check that it's actually there. I think he simply meant the diet he observed in Crete, where he found a very low rate of CVD, and a diet that was rather different to that in the US. But then, he did visit during Lent. He also found the same diet in Corfu, where the rate of CVD was eight times higher.

Do I believe that the Mediterranean diet, whatever it is, is healthy? It is certainly not unhealthy. Salads and olive oil, fish and vegetables, etc., certainly taste nice, especially when eaten outside in the sun with friends and family. However, I also think that all the research in this area is horribly confounded by the fact that, if people think they are eating healthy things, they will be healthy. And healthier people eat things they believe to be healthy.

My own view on diet and health is relatively straightforward and dull. Avoid highly processed foods and eat food that looks like things, e.g. fish or a bit of broccoli, a chicken leg or a tomato. If it takes five minutes to read the list of ingredients on the packet, and it contains more than five ingredients that you have never heard of, then buy something else. I shall call this the Dr Kendrick rule of 'Not eating five unhealthy portions of e numbers'. It is completely arbitrary, just as almost all dietary advice is completely arbitrary.

Moreover, do not eat too many carbs/sugars especially if you are having trouble with weight gain/diabetes. Most of all, enjoy what you eat and, whatever you do, ignore the quite ridiculous 'eat-well' plate and make sure you turn the dietary pyramid upside down.

As for fruit and vegetables – the widely promoted idea that eating five portions of fruit and vegetables is uniquely healthy was never based on any evidence at all. It was, quite simply, made up. If you disagree, here is a challenge. Find the study or studies that the five portions idea was based on. And good luck with that. Many have tried and failed.

CHAPTER 16

Vitamins, Supplements and Medication

⊂⊃

VITAMINS

I must say that I do like vitamins but there is very little good evidence that any vitamin supplement is beneficial. In large part that's because there are not huge profits to be made from selling vitamins, as they cannot be patented.

If a company did a major clinical trial on vitamin K, and found that it saved lives, there would be nothing to stop anyone else selling vitamin K whilst claiming newly discovered health benefits. The company that did the trial would be unable to recoup any research costs. And note, the pharmaceutical industry is doing its level best to attack vitamins as damaging and dangerous, and lobbying madly to have vitamin supplements banned.[1]

Once they achieve this state of Nirvana, they can then invent new synthetic vitamins, patent them and sell them back to us at hugely inflated prices, making massive profits. I just made that bit up, but I wouldn't put it past them. What they are more likely quite legitimately to do is to add vitamins to various other drugs to extent patent life, as Merck was attempting to do with statins and niacin – and failed.

Another problems in trying to get a handle on the potential benefits of vitamins is that it can be very unclear what the optimal dose, or blood levels, might be. This, I believe, is because of the way that vitamins were discovered.

Over many hundreds of years, it was noticed that some diseases occurred when something was missing from the diet. Scurvy was the first of these diseases to be well documented. In 1753 a Scottish surgeon proposed that lemons and limes could prevent and/or cure the condition. Obviously, he had no idea what it was in the limes and lemons that did the trick. Other diseases, such as pellagra and rickets, were then identified as being due to a lack of some substance. The term for these missing substances was 'vital-amines', shortened to vitamins.

It took some time before the vitamins themselves were isolated. The first was vitamin B1 in 1910, the last was vitamin B12 in 1948. There are generally accepted to be 13 vitamins, and many of them are B vitamins of one sort or another. However, in my opinion there are only 12. Vitamin D is really a hormone.

I think vitamin D was only classified as a vitamin because no one knew that it could be synthesised in the skin from sunlight. Whilst people lived mainly outside, there was no vitamin D deficiency, it was only when the industrial revolution started and people began to live and work indoors that rickets (bent, malformed bones) became an epidemic. A lack of vitamin D in the diet was identified as the cause.

Vitamin D looked and acted like a dietary vitamin deficiency, but it was not *actually* a dietary vitamin deficiency. Or, at least, only in part. To prevent rickets, children were given milk. Unfortunately, we are now seeing rickets again because darker skinned Muslim women now fully cover up their skin, and some of them are becoming severely vitamin D depleted.

The reason for this ramble is to make the general point that vitamins were only identified when certain major, immediate and potentially life-threatening illnesses were identified. This meant that the first task was to find the dose, or blood level, that prevented conditions like scurvy, rickets and pellagra. At the time researchers were not looking for longer-term effects, e.g. prevention of CVD, or cancer, etc., so there is no recommended daily allowance that takes optimal health into account.

I sometimes think of the recommended daily intake of vitamins as being just enough to keep you alive but no more. A bit like having a houseplant that is small and shrivelled. But give it some plant feed and it bursts into vigorous growth and is far healthier.

Unfortunately, because we have these hallowed recommended daily intakes, vitamins are viewed by the medical profession as very simple things. You give the vitamin, make sure it gets above a baseline level in the blood and that's that. Nothing to see here, move along.

But if we look at just vitamin B12, the reference (or normal) range is all over the place. In the UK it's set at 110–900ng/l (it's higher in some regions). In the US is it from 200–900ng/l, and in Japan 500–1300ng/l. In Japan and the US, with a level of 110, you would immediately be given additional B12 but in the UK you would be ignored. 'Your level is fine, go away.' I have seen many patients who strongly believe that they need additional Vitamin B12 injections as they feel tired, depressed, etc. The NHS simply ignores them, unless their level is below 110. Perhaps I should advise them to emigrate to Japan.

An additional problem with B12 is that the synthetic B12 normally used is hydroxocobalamin. This is then converted into the active form, methylcobalamin, in the body. However, some people cannot metabolise hydroxocobalamin into methylcobalamin and need methylcobalamin injections, which they cannot get on the NHS. Jolly good. Yes, the more you look into this, the more complicated and frustrating it gets.

Vitamin D is the vitamin most in the news at present. The debate and arguments about it are becoming quite vitriolic. Some doctors refuse to believe that anyone has true vitamin D deficiency, others think that the entire population needs to be dosed with extra amounts during winter. I am very much in the latter group.

For example, it has only recently been discovered that that vitamin D has potent anti-cancer effects, and may reduce the risk of CVD. What level of vitamin D is needed to provide these benefits? Almost certainly a much higher level than that required to prevent rickets. Has this level ever been established? No. What about the risk of developing thin bones in old age? No. Even more recently, a low level of vitamin D has been associated with a much higher level of hospital admission with acute asthma.[2] What level is needed to prevent this happening? No idea. As the potential benefits of vitamin D continue to pile up, the minimum blood level remains unchanged and, it seems, unchangeable.

Now to folate, which, despite its name, is another B vitamin. Folate is known to be essential to prevent neural tube defects in the unborn child, and to produce red blood cells and suchlike. Again, the doses to stop these things happening has not been established.

However, a recent study in Cambridge has shown that B vitamins, including folate, have significant benefits in reducing homocysteine levels, and if you give them in high doses, way above those currently recommended, they may delay or even prevent Alzheimer's disease and reduce or prevent brain shrinkage.[3]

So, what is the correct dose of folate? Enough to stop neural tube defects, or anaemia, or enough to stop Alzheimer's? And can vitamin K prevent atherosclerotic plaques from becoming calcified? Who knows, they have never tested the correct formulation. Can vitamin C reduce the risk of CVD? Who knows? It was tested once in humans, at the wrong dose – at least the wrong dose according to Linus Pauling.

We haven't the faintest clue about the correct doses and blood levels of vitamins required to achieve optimal health. What I do know is that you can take far more than the recommended daily dosage with no problems whatsoever. Vitamins are almost entirely safe. In the US, in 2010, for example, not a single person died from taking a vitamin.[4]

On the other hand, you may be interested to read about the total burden of damage and deaths due to correctly prescribed pharmaceuticals. Read this report from Harvard University:

> Few know that systematic reviews of hospital charts found that even properly prescribed drugs (aside from misprescribing, overdosing, or self-prescribing) cause about 1.9 million hospitalisations a year. Another 840,000 hospitalised patients are given drugs that cause serious adverse reactions for a total of 2.74 million

serious adverse drug reactions. About *128,000 people die from drugs prescribed to them*. This makes prescription drugs a major health risk, ranking 4th with stroke as a leading cause of death. The European Commission estimates that adverse reactions from prescription drugs cause 200,000 deaths; so *together, about 328,000 patients in the US and Europe die from prescription drugs each year*. The FDA does not acknowledge these facts and instead gathers a small fraction of the cases.[5]

So, zero vitamin deaths v 328,000 from drugs per year. If I were looking for something dangerous to ban, it sure as hell would not be vitamins. And which vitamins would I recommend taking? Vitamin D in winter, vitamin C always, along with thiamine and vitamin K2. About five to ten times the recommended daily intake should be fine.

SUPPLEMENTS

What about other supplements, e.g. magnesium, co-enzyme Q10, potassium, L-arginine, L-carnitine, omega-3 fatty acids, etc.? Well I am keen on potassium, very keen. I first noted that higher potassium consumption was associated with significantly reduced mortality in the Scottish Heart Health Study. This was not some minor difference, either. We are talking more than a 50 per cent reduction in overall mortality in men, though less in women.[6] And this was far from an isolated finding. In study after study, potassium reduces blood pressure and, in turn, reduces the risk of CVD and overall mortality.[7] Interestingly, the Mediterranean diet, such as it is, tends to be high in potassium.

As for magnesium – magnesium deficiency is increasingly recognised as a major health issue, and can greatly increase the risk of sudden cardiac death. I now routinely test patients for magnesium levels, as does the rest of the health service, which has belatedly woken up to the importance of this chemical. Magnesium deficiency can also trigger AF, which, in turn, vastly increases the risk of a stroke.[8]

But I feel I am running away with myself. The last thing I want is for people to worry too much about the levels of this and that in the blood. I do not want you rushing to the doctor or a private lab to have everything repeatedly checked.

Take magnesium level deficiency, for example. This is almost unknown if you do not take an acid-lowering drug, such as omeprazole or lansoprazole (both proton pump inhibitors, or PPIs). Unless you are taking one of these, of any other -zole, long term, you are extremely unlikely to be magnesium deficient. As for potassium, get some lo-salt (a mixture of potassium and sodium chloride), or eat lots broccoli and bananas, and you will be fine. Other vegetables are available.

What of omega-3 fatty acids, the fabled fish oil? There is some good quality evidence that they can be good for you. They seem to have beneficial effects on the conduction of electrical impulses in the heart. They are mildly anticoagulant, a bit like aspirin with fewer downsides, such as causing blood loss from the stomach. They also have some benefits on brain function. So, should you take an omega-3 supplement? Easier, I think, to eat fish once a week; sardines on toast is my favourite. But if you feel the need to buy omega-3 supplements, go ahead. The only downside is cost.

A few years ago, I was contacted by a small company that wanted to create a combination pill to reduce the risk of CVD.

They asked me to give them some medical input and support, which I did, but they ran out of money. Before going bust, they did produce a few thousand tubs of Prokardia. A tablet that contained:

- Vitamin K2 12.5µg
- Thiamine 1.7mg
- Folic acid 66.7µg
- Potassium 50mg
- Magnesium 50mg
- L-arginine 600mg
- L-carnitine 50mg
- L-citrulline 16.7mg
- Co-enzyme Q10 33.3mg

The L-arginine and L-citrulline on that list are 'co-factors' for the production of NO in endothelial cells. Co-enzyme Q10 is something I have talked about at some length, and L-carnitine is an amino acid that has been found to have many benefits in CV health. I would have added vitamins D and C to this list, but you can only get so much stuff in one tablet before it becomes a meal in itself.

I would have been more than happy to promote Prokardia as a supplement. It could do no harm, and everything on that list was potentially beneficial for heart health. Unfortunately, Prokardia does not now exist. However, if you took these supplements, in these doses x4 (you were supposed to take four tablets a day), you would not go far wrong.

Having said all this, I do not want everyone to get too carried away with supplements. I have read articles supporting supplement after supplement, and every single vitamin that exists, in high doses. However, it can all get a bit ridiculous. Eat good, natural food and it should be possible to get everything you need from your diet. After all, that was what we were designed to do. Our ancestors did not go around searching for potassium supplements or L-citrulline. It was all there, in the nearest woolly mammoth. All you needed to do was catch it.

MEDICATION

What else might your doctor prescribe? Well, you know my view on statins. How about blood pressure lowering medications? I'd strongly recommend doing everything else possible before taking these, unless your blood pressure is significantly raised to at least 160mmHg systolic.

Even then, before starting on lifelong blood pressure lowering medication, you must try many other things: exercise, weight loss, L-arginine, sunshine, yoga, meditation and increasing potassium consumption. Several people have found that eating the HFLC diet has significant effects on lowering blood pressure. In many cases their blood pressure has returned to normal.

If you have been diagnosed with high blood pressure/ hypertension you need to ensure you are not just suffering 'white coat' hypertension, i.e. increased tension from being surrounded by white-coated doctors. I suggest you buy your own blood pressure monitor and see what your reading is at home, whilst relaxing. It has been estimated that 25 per cent of people are wrongly diagnosed with high blood pressure because they get anxious when they are at the GP's surgery or in hospital. This effect can push the blood pressure very high.

If, having done all of this, your blood pressure remains stubbornly high, get your doctor to check you are not suffering from Conn's syndrome (excess production of aldosterone) and/ or subclinical Cushing's. These conditions are rarely checked for. You will have a battle to get your GP to agree to hunt them down, but Conn's is thought be the cause of a quarter of cases of resistant, raised blood pressure, and subclinical Cushing's is far from rare.

Once you have tried all this, and nothing has worked, you may need to take something to lower the blood pressure. If so, I recommend ACE-inhibitors, first and foremost – all the names end in -pril, as in ramipril, enalapril, etc. They lower blood pressure and increase NO synthesis, which provides a double benefit. In fact, I rather approve of ACE-inhibitors.

However, many people suffer a dry cough if they take an ACE-inhibitor. If so, go for the more modern version, an angiotensin II blocker. These end in -sartan, as is valsartan and irbisartan. If neither ACE-inhibitors or angiotensin II blockers do the trick, try a thiazide diuretic, a blood pressure lowering drug that has been around for ages. I would *not* recommend beta blockers or calcium channel blockers at all. They might lower your blood pressure but can do other things that may cause more harm – particularly the calcium channel blockers.

I say this against a background where more and more people are going to be pressurised into taking tablets. This is because the AHA has created yet another set of guidelines and, guess what, threshold for treatment went up. Ah, no, it has been lowered, yet *again*. Did I hear you say 'inevitably'? They have now decreed that any systolic blood pressure of 130mmHg shall be considered hypertension. This is utterly ridiculous. To quote Richard Lehman in the *BMJ*: 'it reclassifies about half the population as "hypertensive". Here lies a glimmer of hope. *When this level of absurdity is reached*, people might start to question the notion of "hypertension" altogether.'[9] Quite.

What of aspirin? To take or avoid? Aspirin acts as a mild anticoagulant as it interferes with platelets sticking together. It has been proven to be moderately effective at reducing both heart attacks and strokes but the benefits are not hugely impressive, and long-term use can lead to bleeding from the stomach and elsewhere. Again, this risk is small but exists. With aspirin we have small gain and small pain. Would I recommend long-term aspirin use ... probably not, but I could be persuaded.

What I would most definitely warn against, though, is taking a PPI, such as omeprazole, in conjunction with aspirin. This is usually prescribed to protect the stomach from the damaging effects of the aspirin. In fact, the current guidance is to take aspirin and a PPI together, which, as stupid advice goes, is almost up there with sun avoidance.

One of the off-target (pleiotropic) effects of PPIs is to lower NO synthesis. Recent studies have demonstrated that PPIs can *double* the risk of dying of CV, something you would expect once you know what they do to NO production.[10] So, you take aspirin to lower the risk of CVD by around 9 per cent and you take a PPI at the same time, which doubles the risk of CVD. Who, exactly, put these people in charge of anything?

What about preventive mainstream medication? Well, as I said earlier, if you suffer from a specific medical condition, this changes the risk/benefit equation. If, for example, you have AF, then take an anticoagulant, e.g. warfarin, apixaban or rivaroxaban. Absolutely do this, as it massively reduces the risk of a stroke. If you have had a heart attack, take clopidogrel (fancy, expensive aspirin). If you have heart failure, take the medication prescribed.

No, I am not blanket anti-medication, not by any means. What I am against is most preventive medications, prescribed to prevent possible future events. The evidence for any real benefit is vanishingly small to non-existent to, in the case of PPIs, harmful. At the risk of repeating myself, you need to take drugs when something has gone wrong, not before. Clearly, this is not an absolute rule but a good one.

CHAPTER 17

What of Testing and Screening?

W ould you wish to know your future? (Cue spooky music.)
In CV medicine, screening and calculating future risk
has become a vast industry. But should you screen or not? A
very costly CV-screening programme was introduced in the
UK to pick up high blood cholesterol, blood pressure and
early stage diabetes. It now costs several hundred million
pounds per year. When it was analysed, the results were that it
was, and remains, a complete waste of time.[1] So, of course, it
continues.

Unfortunately, and despite repeated failures, the medical
profession is still mesmerised by the idea that if you can pick
up a disease early, and treat it early, all will be well. Superficially,
this seems like pure common sense. Who could object to the
idea? In truth, anyone with a brain. Many things in life are
counter-intuitive, and screening is most certainly one of them.

Before rushing into screening, you need to ask many
questions. For example, is your test remotely accurate? What

percentage of people with the disease does your test correctly pick up? On the other hand, how many people without the disease does it correctly identify as disease-free? No test is 100 per cent accurate. In fact, some are a long way off. Many people are told they have a disease when they do not, and some people who have a disease are missed and given the all-clear.

You also need to ask, is the treatment remotely effective and how much harm might you do in treating people wrongly diagnosed? Also, can screening and scanning change behaviour from the healthy to unhealthy? And finally, for now, can the test itself cause harm? Mammography uses high-dose radiation, with several hundred times as much radiation as a single x-ray. There is a small but recognised risk that it could trigger cancer.

I could go on. The simple fact is that for most types of health screening, when they are assessed objectively, the degree of harm caused can often outweigh the benefits. And that's before you include the enormous amounts of money spent on mass-screening programmes and the resultant opportunity cost, by which I mean what of proven benefit can you *not* do because you have spent so much money on screening?

Despite the growing concerns about screening, if you visit your GP, at some point you will almost certainly end up having your future risk of a CV event calculated. In the UK this is done using an on-line tool called QRISK. We are currently on the third iteration, QRISK3. You feed in various factors, such as age, sex, blood pressure, smoking, LDL level, diabetes, etc., and your chance of suffering a CV event in the next ten years is automatically calculated. You can find the QRISK3 tool at https://qrisk.org/three/. In the US they use the ACC/AHA risk calculator http://www.cvriskcalculator.com/.

The American one is much simpler to use. The main

difference between ACC/AHA and QRISK3 is that the UK version asks about many more factors, such as:

- Chronic kidney disease
- Rheumatoid arthritis
- Systemic lupus erythematosus (SLE)
- Severe mental illness
- Antipsychotic medication? Yes, or no
- Using steroid tablets?
- Diagnosis of erectile dysfunction
- Angina or heart attack in a first-degree relative under the age of 60
- Ethnicity
- Postcode – yes, really

I find this most interesting. At least those asking the questions have finally recognised that many things vastly increase the risk of CVD beyond smoking, blood pressure and raised LDL. About time too, one could say. However, there's no mention *how* these things cause CVD, they just do, and that's that. No more questions, please, or we may have to admit we have no idea what is actually going on.

Whichever system you use, the calculators will use an algorithm to establish your risk of a CV event – fatal and non-fatal – over the next ten years. And they provide a suspiciously accurate percentage figure, e.g. 8.3 or 15.4 per cent risk. In the US, if your risk is over 7.5 per cent you will be put on a statin. In the UK, your official statination figure is a risk greater than 10 per cent. That is, a 10 per cent chance of suffering a CV event in the next ten years.

What you will find, if you play around with the calculators, is that age is by far the most important predictor of them all, especially in the US version. You can set all the other factors to 'perfect' but, as a man, once you reach the age of 60 you will have a risk greater than 10 per cent. Women are officially statinated a few years later. The statination age is obviously lower in the US as they set the treatment risk at 7.5 per cent.

Almost everyone has a slightly increased risk from something else. So, virtually every man will have a risk greater than 7.5 or 10 per cent by their early fifties. You don't need to be a smoker or have diabetes or anything significant, just a slightly raised blood pressure, for example. You can try this out yourself, by moving your figures about. Endless hours of fun for the family. Or maybe not.

Basically, these risk calculators have now decreed that all citizens of the land, man or women, should be taking a statin by the age of – on average – fifty-five. Every single person, for the rest of their lives. And you wonder why I called this book *A Statin Nation*. In the UK, this represents about 15–20 million people, in the US I would imagine we are closer to 200 million.

This is clearly nuts. When you then add in the new AHA guidelines on hypertension, virtually everyone will also be taking blood pressure lowering medication at the same time. Think that's a good thing? After the guidelines on CV risk were changed in the UK, lowering the ten-year event rate from 20 to 10 per cent, the GP conference of the British Medical Association took a vote, where the new guidelines were unanimously rejected. 'Similarly, the Royal College of General Practitioner's official consultation response cited concerns the move would result in 'medicalisation of five million healthy adults' and warned it risked 'the loss of professional confidence in the healthcare targets they are being asked to meet' – pointing to Pulse's finding *that most GPs themselves would not opt to take a statin at this level of risk.*'[2]

Did this vote have any impact? Did it heck. It is amazing how powerless all individuals and organisations are in the face of official medical guidelines. They are carved in stone and handed down to us puny humans by the gods. In truth, guidelines are made up by a bunch of about ten doctors in a room, almost all of whom will have worked closely with the pharmaceutical industry at one time or another. What a surprise.

As for the calculations themselves ... are they remotely accurate? A study in the US found that the ACC/AHA calculator vastly overestimated the figures. A group of researchers looked at the actual number of events that occurred over a five-year period (rather than ten years), and found the following:

- For a predicted risk less than 2.5 per cent, the actual number of events was 0.2 per cent
- For a predicted risk between 2.5 and 3.74 per cent, the actual number of events was 0.65 per cent
- For a predicted risk between 3.75 and 4.99 per cent, the actual number of events was 0.9 per cent
- For a predicted risk equal to or greater than 5 per cent, the actual number of events was 1.85 per cent

'From a relative standpoint, the overestimation is approximately five- to six-fold,' explained Dr Go. 'Translating this, it would mean that we would be over-treating a good many people based on the risk calculator.'[3] Which is what I call masterful understatement – 'a good many people' means hundreds of millions of people who have had their risk vastly overestimated. Quite extraordinary. We might as well stick bones though our noses and leap around in a tent filled with hemp smoke, seeking visions from the gods.

In truth, this is not really news. It has been known for many years that if you use CV risk calculators on different populations they simply do not work. If, for example, you use a US or UK risk calculator on a French population, you must divide whatever figure you obtain by four. Why? The French had/have around one quarter the rate of CVD, with virtually identical risk factors.

This, you would think, might give the researchers pause for thought. Do we really know what causes CVD when we need to incorporate such a massive fudge factor? This is not a few per cent here or there, the fudge factor is four times the size of the total figure you calculated in the first place. If you use the calculator for young Australian aboriginal women, you need to multiply by 30.

Do I think you should pay the slightest attention to the risk calculated for you by the on-line tools? Have a guess.

What of other CV tests? You have probably been offered a scan to see if you have plaques in your carotid arteries at the base of your neck. In addition, you may be offered screening for abdominal aortic aneurysm. There is also a coronary artery calcium (CAC) test and now we have computerised tomography (CT) angiograms. Should you have them done?

These tests can tell you what is going on in your arteries, true. Or at least they can tell you what has happened in the past. Then what? Whilst writing this book a study came out demonstrating that, unless you are suffering an acute MI, there is no point having a stent put into your coronary arteries. It does no good.[4] CABG is no better. So, we do a test to tell you that you have horribly blocked coronary arteries, and then we can do nothing about it. Or nothing useful anyway. So, what was the point in doing the test?

If, on the other hand, you have very clogged carotid arteries in the neck it may possibly be worth having something done, just about. But the blockage must be greater than 50 per cent, and even then it is not clear how beneficial any operation may be. The evidence of benefit is not strong, to say the least.[5] Not only that, but the operation could kill you or trigger a stroke. The risk is not great, but it is far from trivial. The same type of problem exists for abdominal aortic aneurysm (a balloon-like weakness in the aorta). Getting that sorted out is one hell of a major operation that carries a high risk of mortality and illness. Yes, screening can end up killing you as well as potentially saving you.

By now, I hope you may understand more clearly why I am not a great fan of screening, scanning, testing and measuring risk. The tests may or may not accurately define risk (in fact they often don't). And the interventions following the screening may be completely useless, or only marginally effective.

The anxiety created when you are told there is something seriously wrong will be massive. Of course, not all screening is useless but, before you are seduced by a glossy brochure offering you cut-price screening tests, ensure that you do some homework and ask some difficult questions. Screening is always presented as risk-free. It is far from that simple.

BLOOD CLOTTING/THROMBOPHILIA

I have talked quite a lot about blood clotting in this book. It is critically important to the whole process of CVD, but what can you do to reduce the risk? Well, despite what I have said about screening, there are specific conditions such as factor V Leiden and Hughes's syndrome. These are genetic and can greatly increase the risk of CVD. Should you be checked for them? As far as I know the health service has no interest in screening for either of these conditions, so it would have to be done privately. You can find out more at the APS website (http://aps-support.org.uk/). (Hughes's syndrome is also known as antiphospholipid syndrome, or APS.)

As for other clotting factors, can you get screened for a more generally raised thrombophilia risk (i.e. the generally increased risk of blood clots)? As mentioned, thrombophilia can greatly increase stroke and heart attacks. Not only that but it can increase the chance of deep vein thrombosis and therefore a PE. This is another relatively common form of CV death, although this clot forms in the veins in your leg before breaking off and travelling to the lungs. But hey, dead is dead. However, if you want to be screened, again go private.

However, most such screening will almost certainly not look for factors such as plasminogen activator inhibition PAI-1, prothrombin, fibrinogen or increased factor VII, etc. It focuses on established abnormalities.

At present I believe that the only test that is relatively easy to have done and not that expensive is checking your LP(a) level. If it is high then take niacin and high doses of vitamin C to stop Lp(a) having to plug cracks in your arteries, primarily by making sure that you have no cracks to plug.

What else? Omega-3 fatty acids can stop clots forming by reducing platelet stickiness. The Inuit, who traditionally eat a lot of fish, have a very low rate of CVD but they do have a high rate of nose bleeds. A price worth paying? Probably.

In addition, ensure that you keep your NO levels up. You

do this with sunshine, exercise, relaxation, L-arginine and L-citrulline. Also, of course, with Viagra. Recent studies have shown that people with diabetes who take Viagra are three times less likely to die of CVD than men who do not.[6] Yet, weirdly, men with diagnosed CVD are advised *not* to take Viagra. Once again, bonkers.

CHAPTER 18

Heart Rate Variability (HRV)

I t has been known for many years that if you monitor foetal heart rate during labour, the single most important danger sign is a lack of HRV. By which I mean that the normal accelerations and declarations that happen during labour start to disappear, and the tracing begins to look like a flat line. If you see this loss of HRV, get the baby out as fast as you can. It is struggling and may soon die.

Some researchers wondered if a lack of HRV could also be a cause of concern in adults. As people get older, HRV diminishes and it is much more difficult to spot because the accelerations and deceleration in adults are far smaller and more subtle. You need a computer programme to measure the alterations between each heartbeat, and there are plenty of devices out there that can do this.

I like to think of HRV as the heart constantly hunting for the optimal rate, and the greater the flexibility of your CV physiology the more able it is to rapidly speed up and down in response to the hundreds of different signals your heart is getting, every second.

So, does a poor HRV mean anything? Well, there are many conflicting results. Some researchers say that HRV is a vital measure, others dismiss it. The reason why some researchers dismiss it is because raised HRV is closely associated with several other factors that are closely linked to a high risk of CVD. This means that, once you factor them all in, the effect of HRV can be 'explained away' by other things. This, anyway, is the party line. But we immediately run straight into one of the most stupid things that happens in medical research. Possibly *the* most stupid. Which is to treat all risk factors as completely unconnected phenomena.

To explain. We know that HRV is affected by chronic negative stress and short-term acute stress.[1] This is because chronic negative stress damages the neurohormonal system in the body – the flight or fight system, sometimes called the hypothalamic-pituitary-adrenal axis HPA-axis.

We know that once the HPA-axis is dysfunctional, this leads to a series of downstream abnormalities, including central obesity, high blood pressure, raised LDL, raised blood clotting factors and insulin resistance, to name but five. If you find these factors together, this is often referred to as the metabolic syndrome, which is considered the precursor to type 2 diabetes. And the metabolic syndrome is associated with a far higher rate of CVD. However, these five factors do not exist in isolation, they are brought together by negative stress, as outlined in the paper 'The metabolic syndrome –a neuroendocrine disorder?' It says: 'Central obesity is a powerful predictor for disease. By utilizing salivary cortisol measurements throughout the day, it has now been possible to show on a population basis that perceived stress-related cortisol secretion frequently is elevated in this condition. This is followed by insulin resistance, central accumulation of body fat, dyslipidaemia and hypertension (the metabolic syndrome).'[2]

In short, chronic stress damages the neurohormonal system leading to a series of downstream problems. Or, put another way, chronic negative stress is the underlying cause of the metabolic syndrome. However, the party line is to treat the individual abnormalities of the metabolic syndrome as separate and unconnected phenomena. 'Oh look, here is someone with central obesity and, goodness me, they also have raised blood pressure, raised LDL, raised blood clotting factors and – goodness me – insulin resistance *and* raised blood sugar levels. We know that each of these is a cause of CVD. If we add them all together, HRV does not add anything to the calculated increase in risk. Ergo, it is not an important abnormality to measure.'

How sensible is this? Answer, not very.

Having said this, HRV is not a cause of anything either, it is simply a way of measuring a dysfunctional HPA-axis. However, it is a good one because it is non-invasive and simple to do. In 'The metabolic syndrome' paper I just quoted, the impact of chronic stress was measured by taking hourly cortisol levels, over a 24-hour period, which is costly and time consuming and not something you want to be doing on a regular basis.

Instead, you can simply do an HRV measurement, and this will give you a good indication of your overall CV health. Importantly, you can also use the HRV to measure improvements in heart health. The type of things that improve HRV are physical activity, meditation and mindfulness. Yes, all the things you might expect.[3]

Does this improvement in HRV translate into a reduced risk of CVD? Unfortunately, there have not been any major studies, but we do know that if you have poor HRV your risk of CVD is greatly increased. We also know that exercise and mindfulness, etc., improves HRV, as does yoga, which can create significant improvement in the metabolic syndrome. 'Yoga can significantly reduce cardiovascular risk factors including body mass index, blood pressure, and low-density lipoprotein (LDL) cholesterol, says a systematic review that found it had similar benefits to aerobic activities such as cycling or brisk walking.'[4]

You could, of course, say that there is no need to measure HRV at all. Simply do all the things that we know are good for you and your HRV will improve. Yes, this is true, but I do find that most people love a measurement, and they love to see measurements go in the right direction. In my view, if you are going to measure anything, measure HRV.

CHAPTER 19

Salt

I have not mentioned salt yet, but I think it is important because this perfectly innocuous substance has been placed into the same category as cholesterol. A DEADLY KILLER that must not be consumed.

If you go to many schools, they have removed salt cellars from tables lest children commit suicide by sprinkling salt on their food. I have seen this nonsense creeping into restaurants as well, where the salt has been whisked away from the customer. At least McDonald's still allows you pick up a little packet of salt to do with as you will. No skull and crossbones on the packet, yet.

The idea behind the vilification of salt is very simple, and it has been around for many years. It goes like this. If you eat salt, your blood pressure will rise, which will then kill you from strokes and heart disease. Simple, easy to understand ... and wrong.

Yes, if you eat salt your blood pressure does go up, a bit. On average by around 2mmHG. A difference so vanishingly small that you would never even notice it if you checked your own blood pressure. It would be drowned out by day-to-day, hour-to-hour variations. However, on average, if you eat more salt your blood pressure does rise by a smidge. That is true.

On the other hand, if you consume less salt your body triggers a series of other mechanisms to maintain healthy blood pressure. As the pressure drops, the kidneys release aldosterone, the blood pressure raising hormone. This in turn triggers another system into action known as the renin-angiotensin system (RAAS). Simultaneously, the 'stress' sympathetic nervous system is activated to constrict blood vessels and make the heart pump harder and faster.

These are all, as you can probably imagine, potentially damaging to heart health. Let's just focus on one substance that is released when you restrict salt intake, which is angiotensin. This enzyme is quite toxic to the endothelium. It also reduces NO synthesis, which increases the risk of blood clotting.[1] In fact, if you trigger RAAS, there is evidence of significant CVD harm. On the other hand, if you inhibit RAAS, this is highly beneficial. 'Evidence shows that *inhibition* of RAAS positively influences vascular remodelling thus improving CVD outcomes. The beneficial vascular effects of RAAS inhibition are likely due to decreasing vascular inflammation, oxidative stress, endothelial dysfunction, and positive effects on regeneration of endothelial progenitor cells.'[2]

So, reducing salt intake may lower your blood pressure by a small amount but, in turn, it fires up RAAS, a system almost perfectly designed to increase the risk of CVD. And what does the evidence say? Does salt restriction do more good than harm? This is a grey area. There have been almost no controlled studies on lowering salt/sodium intake, and those that have been done have proven little one way or another.[3] In part this is because controlling salt intake, long term, in two different groups of people, is a very difficult thing to do.

Have you, for example, any idea how much sodium you ate yesterday or the day before? I guess you have not the foggiest. Yes, you can sprinkle salt on your food, although I maintain that you have no idea how much you are sprinkling. Do you know what 1g of salt looks like? If so, you are better informed than me. In addition, much of the salt you eat is contained within the food itself and is thus completely hidden.

The other complicating fact is that most research papers talk about sodium and not salt intake. As all budding scientists know salt is NaCl (one sodium atom, one chorine atom). If you eat 1g of salt you will eat 0.5g of sodium (roughly). However, there are other sources of sodium, not attached to chlorine. For example, baking soda – sodium bicarbonate. Also, a number of indigestion medicines contain sodium and no chlorine. Thus, working out the sodium/salt intake is not simple, nor is controlling it.

One man who did manage to do some important work on the effect of reducing salt intake is Michael Alderman. I would like to emphasise that he is not some wild maverick. He was editor of the *American Journal of Hypertension*, a fellow of the American College of Physicians, a member of the Association of American Physicians, and a past president of both the American Society of Hypertension and the International Society of Hypertension.

However, he fell from grace because he changed his mind.

He did a series of studies on patients with heart failure, who, it was thought, would be most affected and most damaged by excess salt intake. In his first study he found that if you reduced salt intake, the mortality rate shot up by 430 per cent.[4]

He repeated the study and got pretty much the same results. He now feels that the war on salt may be rather misguided, to put it mildly. He, along with a few other brave souls, battle against the current dogma where 'experts' belittle and attack anyone who dares to suggest that salt is not a deadly substance.

In 2013 the Institute of Medicine (IOM) did a major review of salt intake and came to the following, somewhat mealy mouthed conclusion: ' [the] Science was insufficient and inadequate to establish whether reducing sodium intake below 2,300mg/d either decreases or increases CVD risk in the general population.'[5]

Alderman followed up this paper with his own exhaustive review of the evidence, and concluded that: 'Our study extends the IOM report by identifying a specific range of sodium intake (2,645–4,945mg) associated with the most favorable health outcomes, within which variation in sodium intake is not associated with variation in mortality. Moreover, this optimal range of intake, based upon available evidence, is coterminous with the current dietary intake of most of the world's population.'[6]

In short, everyone in the world is eating about the right amount of salt to remain healthy, i.e. 2,645–4,945 grams of sodium a day, which is about 6–12g of salt. How harmful is it to eat more or less salt?

We appear to have, with salt intake, what is known as a U-shaped curve, with mortality rising as salt intake drops below about 6g day, and rising at the other end, if salt intake is greater than about 12g a day. Stay between these figures and all is well.

Despite the evidence, the current recommendation is that everyone should eat less than 6g of salt a day. Guidelines which, were they be to be followed, would increase rather than decrease life expectancy. Yet again, the official advice is wrong.

CHAPTER 20

The Placebo Effect

Finally, you may be happy to know that the placebo effect is your friend. If you do *anything*, and I mean virtually *anything*, that you believe to be healthy then it will be good for you. Even if you know it is a placebo.

A number of doctors have been rather worried about the ethics of giving placebos to patients, whilst pretending they are taking an active drug that will have beneficial effects. It turns out that you don't need to pretend at all. You can hand over an inactive substance and say that although it is an inactive substance, taking it *will* make you feel better ... and it does. Ergo, you do not need to lie to patients at all.

This isn't so much the placebo effect as the healthy adherer effect. It seems that whatever someone does – and it doesn't much matter what that something is – and they keep doing it consistently, it will do them good. If you think drinking red wine is good for you, it will be good for you. If you think drinking coffee is good for – keep doing it, it will be great. So read this ...

'Clinicians need to read observational studies reporting surprising benefits of drug therapy with a healthy scepticism. Observational studies of preventive medications and health behaviours are susceptible to various sources of bias, including the so-called healthy-user and healthy-adherer biases. In this article, evidence of the healthy-adherer effect is demonstrated by showing that adherence to statins is associated with a reduction in the risk of accidents (e.g., workplace or motor vehicle), outcomes that would not be expected to be affected by a statin. The approximate magnitude of the adherer effect was a 15% relative risk reduction.'[1]

Ironically, of course, when unexpected benefits are found in statin studies, the researchers jump about claiming that statins can have benefits on such things as cancer. Sorry guys, you could have achieved these benefits with drinking five cups of coffee a day, or slapping your cheeks ten times each morning. Five on the right, followed by five on the left, or vice versa.

Yes, it is the old mind-body connection thing again. So difficult to quantify or research, but so important. A positive, mental attitude. Every day, in every way, things are getting better and better. Have fun, enjoy yourself, know that you are doing yourself some good. This is not new-age, happy-clappy nonsense. It is real, it is powerful, it is important.

In the book *The Blue Zones*, the single most important characteristic of those who lived long, healthy lives was a sense of purpose, a reason for being on the planet. Something positive and life-affirming. However small, however personal. Something to adhere with, something to adhere *for*. Sorry, but there is no blood test for this.

And now we come my list of the ten things you should do to improve your health, and live a long and happy life.

CHAPTER 21

The Top Ten Ways to Avoid Heart Disease and Live Longer

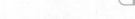

1. Do not smoke
2. Take exercise
3. Spend time in the sun
4. Start doing: yoga/meditation/mindfulness (whichever one floats your boat)
5. Ensure you are connected to the society around you in some way
6. Have a positive mental attitude
7. Eat more fat and less carbohydrate – eat natural foods, do not worry about salt
8. Take a few key supplements
9. Do not worry about your cholesterol level
10. Avoid taking more than five medications – if at all possible.

Finally, I need to add that if you find yourself suffering a worrying/serious symptom, then do go and see your doctor.

Mainstream medicine should *not* be avoided, it should be embraced as it can save your life.

Notes

Introduction

1. http://www.telegraph.co.uk/news/2017/11/15/half-over-65s-take-least-five-drugs-day/

2. http://www.medscape.com/viewarticle/881689#vp_3

3. http://www.dietsdontwork.co.uk/sweden-rejects-low-fat

4. https://www.theguardian.com/society/2016/jan/08/tough-drinking-guidelines-not-scaremongering-says-chief-medical-officer

5. https://www.spectator.co.uk/2009/07/to-become-an-extremist-hang-around-with-people -you-agree-with/

6. Meador, C., 'The Last Well Person', *NEJM*, 10 February 1994, pp. 400-1

7. http://www.medscape.com/viewarticle/460474_5

8. ACCORD – Action to Control Cardiovascular Risk in Type II Diabetes; the study is at http://www.nejm.org/doi/full/10.1056/NEJMoa0802743#t=abstract

9. 'The impact of differing glucose lowering regimens on the pattern of association between glucose control and survival', 2018: http://onlinelibrary.wiley.com/doi/10.1111/dom.13155/epdf

10. https://en.wikipedia.org/wiki/Procrustes

Chapter 1 What is CVD?

1. Newsletter of the American Institute of Stress, vol. 12, Dec 2008

Chapter 3 What is Atherosclerosis?

1. https://www.ncbi.nlm.nih.gov/pubmed/25769003

2. https://www.ncbi.nlm.nih.gov/pubmed/26714212

3. http://advances.nutrition.org/content/3/2/158.long

Chapter 4 Heart Attacks and Strokes

1. Sun Y, Weber T., 'Infarct scar: a dynamic tissue', *Cardiovascular Research* 46, 2000, pp. 250–6

2. http://heart.bmj.com/content/96/18/1434

3. http://www.nytimes.com/1984/07/22/obituaries/james-f fixx-dies-jogging-author-on-running-was-52.html

4. https://www.ncbi.nlm.nih.gov/pmc/articles/PMC4677871/

5. 'Stroke prevention in atrial fibrillation study. Final results', *Circulation*, 1991; 84: pp. 527–39

Chapter 5 What are Fats?

1. https://www.westonaprice.org/health-topics/know-your-fats/the-tragic-legacy-of-center-for-science-in-the-public-interest-cspi/

Chapter 6 Triglycerides

1. https://www.ncbi.nlm.nih.gov/books/NBK22436/

2. https://www.ncbi.nlm.nih.gov/pubmed/28030918

Chapter 7 What is Cholesterol?

1. http://www.cholesterol-and-health.com/Cholesterol-Cell-Membrane.html

2. http://thescipub.com/abstract/10.3844/ojbsci.2014.167.169

3. https://www.ncbi.nlm.nih.gov/pmc/articles/PMC2900496/

Chapter 8 What is Your Blood Cholesterol Level?

1. http://www.fiercebiotech.com/r-d/failure-of-lilly-s-evacetrapib-may-prove-final-nail-coffin-for-cetp

2. http://www.reuters.com/article/us-health-cholesterol-idUSKCNOWC2HI

3. Gresele, P. (ed), *Platelets in Thrombotic and Non-Thrombotic Disorders*, Cambridge University Press, 2002, p.5

4. https://www.ncbi.nlm.nih.gov/pmc/articles/PMC1823880/?page=3

5. https://www.ncbi.nlm.nih.gov/pmc/articles/PMC3295201/

6. http://pulmccm.org/main/2017/critical-care-review/vitamin-c-save-lives-sepsis/

7. *See* Iribarren, C., et al., 'Cohort study of-serum total cholesterol and in-hospital incidence of infectious diseases', *Epidemiology and Infection*, 1998; 121(2): pp 335-47.

8. http://www.jci.org/articles/view/118556/pdf

9. https://www.ncbi.nlm.nih.gov/pubmed/26392394

10. https://www.ncbi.nlm.nih.gov/pmc/articles/PMC31037/

11. http://bmjopen.bmj.com/content/6/6/e010401

12. https://www.ncbi.nlm.nih.gov/pmc/articles/PMC4344393/

13. Rath, M., Niendorf, A., Tjark Reblin, T., et al., 'Detection and Quantification of Lipoprotein(a) in the Arterial Wall of 107 Coronary Bypass Patients', *Arteriosclerosis* 9, September/October 1989, pp. 579–92

Chapter 9 Cholesterol Lowering Without Statins

1. http://www.pmlive.com/pharma_news/cetp_inhibitor_class_finally_dies_as_merck_abandons_anacetrapib_1208239

2. https://www.forbes.com/sites/matthewherper/2015/10/12/eli-lillys-good-cholesterol-drug-goes-bad/#47d83c527de8

3. http://www.mdedge.com/ecardiologynews/article/108182/lipid-disorders/accelerate-evacetrapibs-clinical-failure-sinks-lipid

4. https://www.ncbi.nlm.nih.gov/pubmed/2861880

5. http://www.thennt.com/nnt/anti-hypertensives-for-cardiovascular-prevention-in-mild-hypertension/

6. https://www.ncbi.nlm.nih.gov/pubmed/6863470

7. http://www.jlr.org/content/47/1/1.full

8. http://www.nytimes.com/2008/01/14/business/14cnd-drug.html

9. http://www.bmj.com/rapid-response/2011/11/02/failure-enhance-trial-time-evidence-based-medicine-step

10. http://drnevillewilson.com/2008/02/04/the-enhance-trial-its-failure-concerns/

11. http://www.medscape.com/viewarticle/814152

12. https://www.ncbi.nlm.nih.gov/pmc/articles/PMC2292314/

13. http://www.ahjonline.com/article/S0002-8703(10)00227-9/pdf

14. http://www.nejm.org/doi/pdf/10.1056/NEJMoa1410489

15. https://clinicaltrials.gov/archive/NCT00202878/2015_09_29/changes

16. http://www.medscape.com/viewarticle/835030#vp_2

17. https://www.reuters.com/article/us-merck-zetia-fda/merck-fails-to-win-fda-panel-backing-for-vytorin-heart-claim-idUSKBN0TX2IL20151214

18. http://www.thelancet.com/journals/lancet/article/PIIS0140-6736(15)60696-1/fulltext

19. https://www.ncbi.nlm.nih.gov/pmc/articles/PMC4572812/

20. http://www.thelancet.com/pdfs/journals/lancet/PIIS0140-6736%2815%2960696-1.pdf

21. https://blogs.bmj.com/bmj/2014/01/31/richard-smith-medical-research-still-a-scandal/

22. http://www.npr.org/sections/health-shots/2017/05/09/527575055/one-third-of-new-drugs-had-safety-problems-after-fda-approval

23. https://www.ncbi.nlm.nih.gov/pubmed/?term=24449315

24. http://blogs.sciencemag.org/pipeline/archives/2017/04/27/a-clinical-trial-torpedoed-by fraud-and-incompetence

25. http://www.bmj.com/content/346/bmj.f707

26. https://en.wikipedia.org/wiki/Marcia_Angell

27. http://www.bmj.com/content/353/bmj.i2412

28. https://www.thelancet.com/journals/lancet/article/PIIS0140-6736(15)60696-1/fulltext

29. http://www.investopedia.com/terms/b/blockbuster-drug.asp

30. https://heartuk.org.uk/fh-familial-hypercholesterolemia/children-and-familial-hypercholesterolaemia-fh

31. https://www.ncbi.nlm.nih.gov/pmc/articles/PMC1853359/

32. http://www.bbc.co.uk/news/health-27586009

33. http://circ.ahajournals.org/content/133/11/1054

34. https://www.bhf.org.uk/heart-health/conditions/familial-hypercholesterolaemia

35. http://www.bmj.com/content/344/bmj.e3863

36. http://www.medscape.com/viewarticle/877348#vp_1

Chapter 10 What is a Statin?

1. http://www.webmd.com/cholesterol-management/side-effects-of-statin-drugs#1

2. https://www.nature.com/articles/srep00679

3. https://www.ncbi.nlm.nih.gov/pubmed/16614729

4. https://www.ncbi.nlm.nih.gov/pmc/articles/PMC3309426/

5. http://www.onlinejacc.org/content/accj/46/8/1425.full.pdf

6. Ibid.

7. http://road.cc/content/news/68212-dft-casualty-statistics-rank-driving-cycling-walking-and-motorcycling-risk

8. http://www.jpands.org/vol20no2/miller.pdf

9. http://bmjopen.bmj.com/content/5/9/e007118

10. https://www.cttcollaboration.org/about2

11. http://www.cochrane.org/

12. http://www.ti.ubc.ca/2010/10/18/do-statins-have-a-role-in-primary-prevention-an-update/

13. http://www.nature.com/news/registered-clinical-trials-make-positive-findings-vanish-1.18181

14. https://www.ncbi.nlm.nih.gov/pmc/articles/PMC4513492/

15. http://www.nejm.org/doi/full/10.1056/NEJMsa065779#t=article

16. Maia Szalavitz, 'How Drug Companies Distort Science',Q&A with Ben Goldacre, *Time Magazine*, 28 February 2013: http://healthland.time.com/2013/02/28/how-drug-companies-distort-science-qa-with-ben-goldacre/

Chapter 11 The Downside of Statins

1. http://www.natureworldnews.com/articles/21262/20160427/high-cholesterol-levels-lower-risk-colorectal-cancer.htm

2. https://www.ncbi.nlm.nih.gov/pubmed/11129127

3. https://www.ncbi.nlm.nih.gov/pubmed/9811154

4. https://www.ncbi.nlm.nih.gov/pmc/articles/PMC59524/

5. http://www.nejm.org/doi/full/10.1056/NEJMoa0807646#t=article

6. http://ebm.bmj.com/content/20/4/121.long

7. http://www.medscape.com/viewarticle/840884?pa=UPpaEll4Oof8TDzu-zoZP2SE%2BX
   Aupaa%2FXN6Y%2FKTRjWDmxevOPaeoLz0aNAHHhiw8SlvI8zjYv73GUyW5rsbWA%3D%
   3D

8. https://www.ncbi.nlm.nih.gov/pubmed/17536877

9. https://bernardlown.wordpress.com/2012/11/03/power-to-the-people-patient-in-
   command/

10. http://www.cardiobrief.org/2017/07/24/nissen-calls-statin-denialism-a-deadly-
    internet-driven-cult/

11. http://www.statinusage.com/Pages/about-survey-respondents.aspx

12. https://www.medicalnewstoday.com/articles/317931.php

13. https://www.sciencedaily.com/releases/2013/01/130103114211.htm

14. https://academic.oup.com/brain/article/130/8/2037/307340

15. https://www.ncbi.nlm.nih.gov/pubmed/25655639

16. http://www.statinusage.com/Pages/key-findings-and-implications.aspx

17. https://spacedoc.com/articles/dolichols-vital-to-cell-function

18. https://www.medicalnewstoday.com/articles/317931.php

19. https://www.peoplespharmacy.com/2015/03/16/statins-sap-sex-drive-and-lower-
    testosterone/

Chapter 12 The Diet-Heart Meme

1   http://jaoa.org/article.aspx?articleid=2646761

2. https://www.ncbi.nlm.nih.gov/pubmed/11157321

3. http://www.telegraph.co.uk/news/2016/09/13/sugar-industry-began-blaming-heart-
    disease-on-fat-as-early-as-1964

4. https://www.theguardian.com/society/2016/apr/07/the-sugar-conspiracy-robert-
    lustig-john-yudkin

5. https://therussells.crossfit.com/2017/01/05/big-food-vs-tim-noakes-the-final-crusade/

6. https://www.medscape.com/view-article/884937#vp_3

7. https://research-doc.credit-suisse.com/docView?language=ENG&source=ulg& format=PDF&document_id=1053247551&serialid=MFT6JQWS%2B4FvvuMD-BUQ7v9g4cGa84%2Fgpv8mURvaRWdQ%3D

8. https://www.ncbi.nlm.nih.gov/pmc/articles/PMC5174149/

9. https://www.rippehealth.com/index.htm

10. http://jaoa.org/article.aspx?articleid=2646761

11. http://diabetestimes.co.uk/big-interview-dr-david-unwin/

12. http://www.diabesityinpractice.co.uk/media/content/_master/4311/files/pdf/dip4-3-102-8.pdf

13. http://www.nofructose.com/gary-fettke/

Chapter 13 Does Raised Cholesterol (LDL) Cause CVD?

1. https://www.pcrm.org/media/news/physicians-committee-sues-usda-and-dhhs

2. http://jn.nutrition.org/content/128/2/439S.full

3. https://www.health.harvard.edu/heart-health/ldl-cholesterol-low-lower-and-lower-still

4. https://rarediseases.info.nih.gov/diseases/5683/smith-lemli-opitz-syndrome

5. Ueshima, H., 'Explanation for the Japanese Paradox: Prevention of Increase in Coronary Heart Disease and Reduction in Stroke', *Journal of Atherosclerosis and Thrombosis*, 2007; 14: pp. 278–86

6. Benfante, R., 'Studies of CVD and cause-specific mortality trends in Japanese-American men living in Hawaii and risk factor comparisons with other Japanese populations in the Pacific region: a review', *Human Biology*, 1002; 64: pp. 791–805

7. http://onlinelibrary.wiley.com/doi/10.1111/j.1365-2753.2011.01767.x/pdf

8. https://www.ncbi.nlm.nih.gov/pubmed/21160131

9. http://bmjopen.bmj.com/content/6/6/e010401

10. 'Cholesterol and mortality: 30 years of follow-up from the Framingham Study', *JAMA*, 24 April 1987, pp. 2176–80

11. http://health-heart.org/eve-not-adam.pdf

12. http://journals.plos.org/plosone/article?id=10.1371/journal.pone.0063416

13. https://www.ncbi.nlm.nih.gov/pubmed/19081406

14. http://www.bmj.com/content/346/bmj.e8707

15. http://www.cbc.ca/news/health/saturated-fat-diet-heart-hypothesis-1.3532509

16. http://www.bmj.com/content/353/bmj.i1246

17. https://www.bhf.org.uk/publications/statistics/cvd-stats-2015

18. https://www.ncbi.nlm.nih.gov/pmc/articles/PMC1671226/?page=4

19. Harlan, W., et al, 'Familial Hypercholesterolemia: a genetic and metabolic study', *Medicine*, 1966, Vol. 45, No. 2.

20. https://academic.oup.com/eurheartjarticle/29/21/2625/530400/Reductions-in-all-cause-cancer-and-coronary

21. https://www.ncbi.nlm.nih.gov/pubmed/8551820

22. http://www.thecardiologyadvisor.com/chd/familial-hypercholesterolemia-chd-ascvd-risks/article/506653/

23. https://www.ncbi.nlm.nih.gov/pmc/articles/PMC481754/?page=1

24. http://www.sciencedirect.com/science/article/pii/S0735109797001290#FIG1

25. https://www.ncbi.nlm.nih.gov/pmc/articles/PMC4272949/

Chapter 14 How to Avoid Dying of CVD and Anything Else

1. http://onlinelibrary.wiley.com/doi/10.1111/dom.13155/epdf

2. https://www.ncbi.nlm.nih.gov/pubmed/28540438

3. https://www.ncbi.nlm.nih.gov/pubmed/28899661

4. http://www.independent.co.uk/news/uk/home-news/pensioners-uk-life-expectancy-falling-institute-and-faculty-of-actuaries-a7661571.html

5. http://journals.plos.org/plosmedicine/article?id=10.1371/journal.pmed.1001335

6. Garland, C. et al., 'Vitamin D for Cancer Prevention: Global Perspective', *Annals of Epidemiology* 2009, 19, pp. 468–83

7. http://www.thelancet.com/journals/lancet/article/PIIS0140-6736%2804%2915649-3/fulltext

8. https://www.ncbi.nlm.nih.gov/pubmed/19519827

9. https://www.ncbi.nlm.nih.gov/pubmed/15687362

10. https://www.ncbi.nlm.nih.gov/pmc/articles/PMC1470481/

11. https://www.karger.com/Article/Fulltext/441266

12. https://www.ncbi.nlm.nih.gov/pubmed/26992108

13. https://academic.oup.com/jnci/article/97/3/161/2544132